the total
dumbbell workout

TRADE SECRETS OF A PERSONAL TRAINER

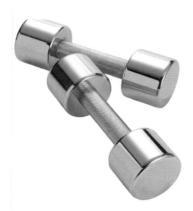

Note

Whilst every effort has been made to ensure that the content of this book is as technically accurate and as sound as possible, neither the author nor the publishers can accept responsibility for any injury or loss sustained as a result of the use of this material.

Published by Bloomsbury Publishing Plc
49–51 Bedford Square, London WC1B 3DP
www.bloomsbury.com

First edition 2011

ISBN 978 1 4081 4228 8

10 9 8 7 6 5 4 3

A CIP catalogue record for this book is available from the British Library.

Acknowledgements
Cover photographs © Grant Pritchard, central image © Shutterstock
Inside photographs: All inside photographs © Grant Pritchard with the exception of the following: pp. 1, 5–7, 9, 11–2, 16, 20, 32, 38, 41, 55, 69, 71–2, 77, 93, 107, 109, 114, 120 © Shutterstock; pp. 14, 22, 27, 36, 103 courtesy and Copyright © of Escape Fitness Ltd.
Illustrations by David Gardner
Designed by James Watson
Commissioned by Charlotte Croft
Edited by Kate Wanwimolruk

This book is produced using paper that is made from wood grown in managed, sustainable forests. It is natural, renewable and recyclable. The logging and manufacturing processes conform to the environmental regulations of the country of origin.

Typeset in 10.25pt on 13.5pt URWGroteskLig by Margaret Brain, Wisbech

Printed and bound in India by Replika Press Pvt. Ltd.

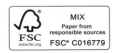

the total
dumbbell workout

TRADE SECRETS OF A PERSONAL TRAINER

STEVE BARRETT

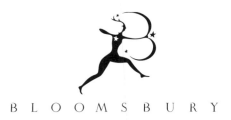

BLOOMSBURY

disclaimer and advisory

Before attempting any form of exercise, especially that which involves lifting weights, always ensure you have a safe working environment. Ensure that the floor surface you are on is non-slip and do not stand on any rugs or mats that could move when you exercise. Also, clear your exercise space of items that could cause you harm if you collided with them; this includes furniture, pets and children. Pay particular attention to the amount of clearance you have above your head and remember that for some of the exercise moves you will be raising your hands and the weights above head height, so keep away from doorways and light fittings.

The information, workouts, health related information and activities described in this publication are practiced and developed by the author and should be used as an adjunct to your understanding of health and fitness and, in particular, strength training. While physical exercise is widely acknowledged as being beneficial to a participant's health and well-being, the activities and methods outlined in this book may not be appropriate for everyone. It is fitness industry procedure to recommend all individuals, especially those suffering from disease or illness, to consult their doctor for advice on their suitability to follow specific types of activity. This advice also applies to any person who has experienced soft tissue or skeletal injuries in the past, those who have recently received any type of medical treatment or are taking medication and women who are, or think they may be, pregnant.

The author has personally researched and tried all of the exercises, methods and advice given in this book, on himself and with many training clients. However, this does not mean these activities are universally appropriate and neither he nor the publishers are, therefore, liable or responsible for any injury, distress or harm that you consider may have resulted from following the information contained in this publication.

contents

1 the basics of exercising with dumbbells

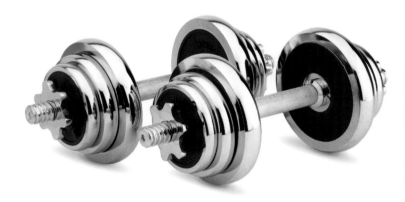

the S.A.F.E. trainer system
(Simple, Achievable, Functional, Exercise)

. . . .

We need to exercise our bodies in a way that is achievable, effective and, most of all, sustainable so that the method becomes part of our lifestyle, rather than an inconvenience.

In a perfect world everyone would be able to lift their own body weight above their head, have ideal body fat levels and be able to run a four-minute mile. Any one of these goals is achievable if you are highly motivated and have very few other commitments in your life, but the reality is that most 'real people' are so far off this state of perfection that the biggest challenge is either starting an exercise programme, or staying committed and engaged with a method of training for long enough to see any kind of improvement.

Exercise is in many ways a perfect product because it has very few negative side effects, it is cheap to do and highly versatile. But so many high profile, quick-fix programmes and products make exercise sound easy, as though it is a magic wand that once waved will bring near instant results. And with the fitness industry constantly driven by innovation in products and methods, the diverse and sometimes bewildering amount of advice available makes it all too easy to be overwhelmed. The truth is that many training programmes and methods will theoretically work, but the level of commitment needed is so high that when you add in work and family responsibilities, stress and other demands upon time, most of us simply cannot stick to a plan.

I also find that those programmes which seem too good to be true usually have a series of components that are not explicit in the headline, but are required to achieve the spectacular results it boasts about. So you sign up to a workout programme claiming: 'Instant fat loss – ultra 60 second workout!' only to find that to achieve the promised weight loss you have to go on an impossible 500 calorie a day diet. These methods also assume that everybody is fairly perfect already; by this I mean they don't have any injuries, they are strong, mobile and flexible and have a cardiovascular system that will soak up anaerobic training from day one. If these people are out there I don't see them walking up and down the average high street. There is a real need to approach fitness in a more down

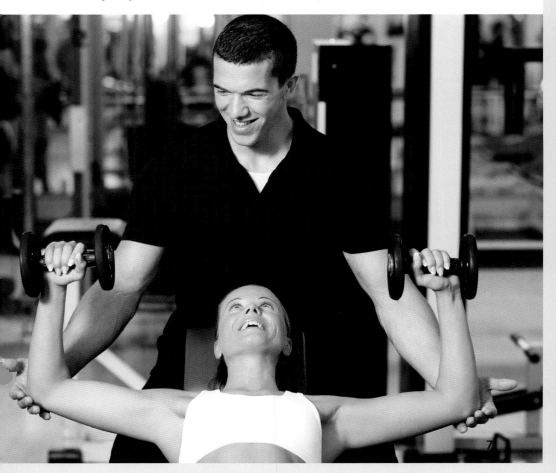

. . . .

to earth, less sensationalist way. We need to exercise our bodies in a way that is achievable, effective and, most of all, sustainable so that the method becomes part of our lifestyle, rather than an inconvenience.

My S.A.F.E. trainer system (Simple, Achievable, Functional, Exercise) is all of these things. It is based on 20 years of personal training experience, including many thousands of hours of coaching, lifting, running, jumping and stretching with people from all walks of life, from the average man or woman to elite athletes. My system respects the natural way that the body adapts to activity and creates a perfect physiological learning curve.

All S.A.F.E. trainer system moves develop stability, strength or power. If you're not familiar with these essential components of human performance, I am sure that you will recognise the saying: 'You have to walk before you can run'. This is the epitome of my approach, because when a client says they want to run or jump, the first thing I have to establish as a personal trainer is that they are at least already at the walking stage. I consider stability to be the walking phase of human movement, as it teaches you the correct muscle recruitment patterns; strength the running phase, as it trains the body to do these moves against a greater force (resistance); and power the jumping phase, since it teaches you to add speed and dynamics to the movement.

Whether you are a personal trainer, sportsperson or fitness enthusiast, I hope this book will fully equip you to get the most out of the valuable time you spend working out with dumbbells. Dumbbells are an iconic piece of fitness equipment and they offer so many solutions to so many different training objectives. The possibilities are endless, and no matter what your goals, dumbbells can play a significant part in helping you achieve them. This book contains a collection of ideas and observations that I have practiced and developed during two decades as a personal trainer. The reality is many books and guides are written with an attitude that readers have the same commitment and potential ability that professional sportspeople and athletes have. However, the reality is that for many people 'exercise' (the time spent exerting themselves) plays a relatively small part in busy lives and therefore quality of movement and my sensible approach to intensity ensures that rather than simply 'draining' the body, all the exercises you perform with dumbbells will have a positive productive end result.

When you get to the portfolio of exercises (see page 39) demonstrating the actual exercises (or 'moves' as I like to call them) you will find that, rather than just being a list of exercises with dumbbells, I have focused on the moves that really work. There are hundreds of moves that can be done with weights, but many of them are very similar to each other, ineffective or potentially dangerous. This book is all about combining skills and methods to create safe and effective fitness ideas for lifting weights.

You will see that I have given each move a classification: 'isolation', 'integration' and even those worthy of being filed under 'don't waste your time'. Isolation moves are generally good, but are in some ways a luxury, first, because working the body one muscle at a time takes longer than most people have available for a training session and, second, isolation moves do not really mimic the way we ask our body to work day to day. Integration moves are all the exercises that mimic the way we move in everyday life where multiple joints moves with muscles throughout the body play a role either in creating the actual movement or stabilising sections of the skeleton as you move. I included the 'don't waste your time section' because those exercises that are either pointless or potentially dangerous never seem to die. I think this is often because many people learn their technique from watching other people in the gym and replicating their bad habits, rather than getting a proper grounding in how to perform these moves. Therefore, I'm hoping that by including these problem exercises you will realise that some of the 'old favourites' should be laid to rest.

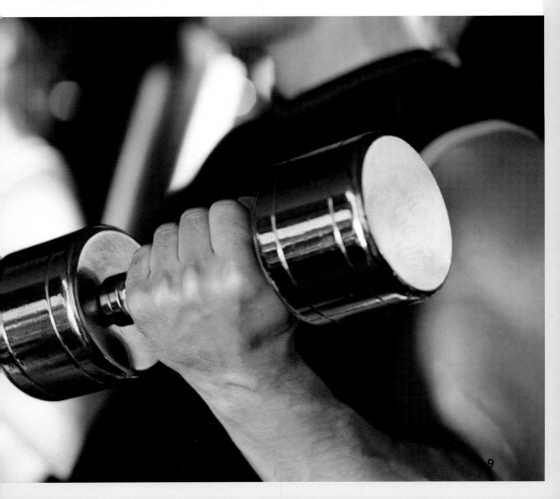

how to use this book

To help you make sense of each dumbbell activity and how it relates to my S.A.F.E. training system, each move is classified by its respective outcome, whether that be an increase in stability, strength or power, rather than the less subjective easy, medium and hard.

In everyday life when we carry out activities that require strength it is through the hands and feet that the majority of force first enters the body (kinetic chain) and therefore challenging muscles and loading the skeleton by using dumbbells is probably the most user friendly and effective way of getting results. Obviously, the amount of time you spend lifting weights will dictate the outcome of your training as will the weight you use, but the actual moves you perform will be the most significant factor for success. The portfolio of moves has been created to ensure that wherever possible, one exercise can be performed to achieve multiple positive results. All the workout sessions are progressive and have been created with the attitude that you can solely use these programmes to provide you with the strength component necessary for a healthy active lifestyle.

When I started to think about writing a book about exercising with dumbbells, the first thing I had to come to terms with is that there are many other books available that set out to teach you how to use dumbbells. Likewise, in my everyday life as a personal trainer I know that my clients have access to information not only from myself, but from a wide range of sources such as the web, books and no doubt other personal trainers they come across in the gym.

As I have worked with many of my clients now for over a decade, clearly they find my approach productive and a worthwhile investment. With this in mind, my aim is to condense 25 years' experience of training my own body and, more importantly, 20 years' experience as a personal trainer and many thousands of hours of training the bodies of other people into this book.

Don't worry: this isn't an autobiography in which I wax lyrical about the celebrities and Premier League footballers I've trained. Yes, I have trained those types of people, but to me every client has the same goal for every training session: they want to get maximum results from the time they are prepared to invest in exercise. Every exercise I select for their session, therefore, has to have earned its place in the programme and every teaching point that I provide needs to be worthwhile and have a positive outcome. In essence, my teaching style could almost be described as minimalist. Now that the fitness industry enters its fourth decade, many of you will have accumulated a level of knowledge and information equal to some fitness professionals in the industry, so I don't go in for trying to show you how clever I am when all that is required are clear and concise instructions.

I learned this lesson many years ago when I was hired as personal trainer to a professor of medicine. There was absolutely nothing I could say about the function of the body that she didn't already know, but what I could do was assess her current level of ability and take her on the shortest, safest and most effective route to an improved level of fitness. Fifteen years on I am still finding new ways to help her enjoy and benefit from the time we spend training together.

The thought process and methods I use are based on my belief that everybody feels better when they build activity into their lives, but not everybody has the motivation and time to create the type of bodies we see on the covers of fitness magazines. When training my clients, I am ultimately judged on the results I deliver. These results can present themselves in many ways, for example, in the mirror or on the weighing scales, but I also aim to help my clients make sense of what we are doing together. I find when talking about any activity it is best to focus on the outcomes rather than use subjective classifications, such as beginner/advanced, easy/hard. Therefore, to help you make sense of each dumbbell activity and how it relates to my S.A.F.E. training system, each move is classified by its respective outcome, whether that be an increase in stability, strength or power, rather than the less subjective easy, medium and hard.

every body is different

Just to be clear, any attempt to classify physical activity has to respect the fact that each human body responds to physical demands differently – there isn't an exact point where one moves stops being beneficial for stability and switches over to being purely for strength. The transition is far more subtle and means that no matter which version of a move you are doing, you will never be wasting your time.

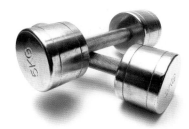

don't skip the moves

Human nature might lead you to think that the way to achieve the quickest results would be to skip the stability and strength moves and start on day one with the power versions. Overcoming this instinct is the fundamental difference between the 'old school approach' of beating up the body every training session, rather than using your training time wisely. My approach is about quality and not quantity. For a personal trainer to take this approach it requires true confidence and belief in the system, as some clients (particularly men) feel that they should be 'working hard' every session. This I feel is a situation unique to fitness training. In no other sport or activity would you set out to teach the body to cope with a new skill or level of intensity by starting with the high intensity or fastest version. For example, if you are learning to play golf, you don't start by trying to hit the ball a long way, rather you start by simply trying to make contact and hit it in the right direction. Or how about tennis? When learning to serve, if all you do is hit the ball as hard as you can, it is unlikely that any shot will ever stay within the lines of the court and therefore count. In all cases quality and the development of skill is the key to success.

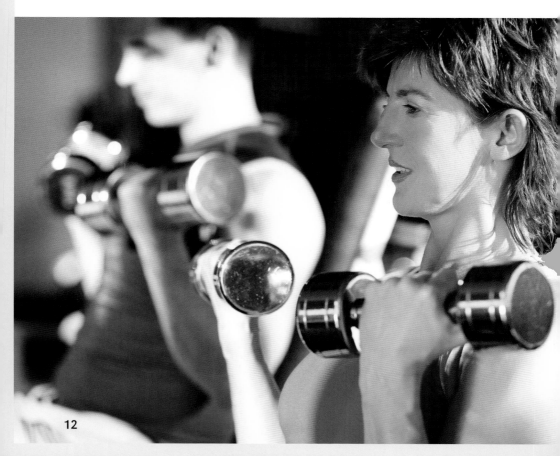

mixing it up

Personal trainers, coaches and instructors think very differently about exercise and human movement today compared to just 10 years ago. In just one decade the focus went from training with dumbbells through limited planes of motion and on machines that moved in straight lines to trying to incorporate the body's three planes of motion (sagittal, transverse and frontal) into the majority of our exercises using both improved weight machines, 'compound' free weight exercises (page 147) and the huge selection of functional training products now available: sagittal involves movements from left to right of the body's centre line; frontal (coronal) involves movements which are forward and backward from the centre line and transverse which are movements that involve rotation. The reality is these planes of motion never occur independently of each other so the best way to ensure you are working through all three planes is to create exercises that incorporate bending and twisting rather than concentrating on movement of joints in isolation. Before functional training equipment (such as the gym ball) became popular we used resistance machines in the gym to help us work muscles in isolation and then relied on the work with free weights (dumbbells and barbells) to do the compound or integrated moves. Isolation moves are generally good for overloading and challenging an individual muscle to adapt and react to the challenges of exercise, but working muscles one at a time leaves you with a body full of great individual muscle when what you actually need are muscles that work as a team and in conjunction with the muscles that surround them. For example, despite most of the classic free weight exercises being integrated movements (i.e. they work more than one set of muscles at a time), the vast majority of free weight moves involve no rotation of the spine (through the transverse plane) and therefore don't train the body for the reality of every day where we constantly rotate at the same time as bending, pushing or pulling against external forces.

As any good personal trainer will tell you, if you only ever do one type of training you will probably miss out on reaching your full potential, so try also to incorporate other types of activity into your week. Many of the moves that follow in this book are to be performed in the prone position (lying face up), so while they are highly productive, it is wise to make them a part of your active lifestyle rather than relying on them to be your single dominant form of exercise. Therefore, I suggest that every session you spend lifting weights you should also try to build in time for upright free-flowing activity, such as walking, jogging or running.

the workouts

In the final section of the book you will find a series of workouts. They are designed to be realistic sessions that you can do on any day of the week, without the need for 'rest' days or anything more than a reasonable amount of space.

All the workouts are sequential, so in theory you could start with 15 minutes of stability moves and do every workout until you reach 45 minutes of power moves. This is, of course, the theory; in reality you will naturally find the right start point depending on how you do with the assessment (see 'Assess, don't guess' on page 21) and how much time you have available on a given day. Continue using that particular workout until you feel ready to move on. I would advise everybody to start with the stability sessions, then move onto strength and then finally power, but I also accept that some people will find that the stability and strength moves don't challenge them enough so they will dive into the power phase. Please bear in mind that, if this is how you plan on approaching the exercises in this book, you might be missing out on a valuable learning curve that the body would benefit from, as well as risking the loss of potential conditioning of some of the less significant muscles that play a key role in many of the more intense exercises.

a resource for life

My aim is for this book to be an ongoing reference point, and I suggest reading the entire contents and then dipping into the specific areas that interest you, such as the training programmes or fitness glossary. I guarantee you'll discover nuggets of information that perhaps you knew a little about, but had never fully understood because they had been explained in such a way that left you confused. If fitness training is an important part of your life, or even your career, then I know this book will be a long-term resource and will help you get the most from the time you spend using dumbbells.

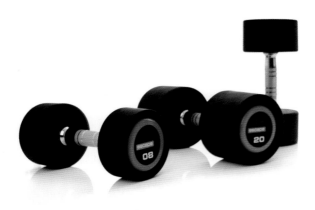

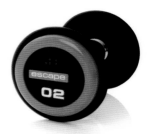

FAQs

When learning to train with dumbbells, there are a handful of important questions that you should ask before attempting to lift the weights. Find the answers here.

What size dumbbells do I need?

This comes down to budget as much as ability. Most people find that they can use heavier weights for the leg exercises than they can most upper body moves, so if you only want to buy one pair of dumbbells, then purchase an adjustable set. It is preferable to have at least two different weights for the upper body. Select the lighter weight for moves that use individual muscles, such as the deltoid raise or triceps press, and then use the heavier weight for moves that use multiple muscle groups, such as the chest press and clean and press. Your heaviest weights will be used for legs exercises.

You will find that if you lift weights frequently your ability will rapidly progress, making exact recommendations subjective.

- For healthy females who are non-athletes, I use a range of 3–7.5kg for upper body work and 7.5–10kg for lower body work.
- For healthy men who are non-athletes, I select from 5–12.5kg for the upper body and 7.5–20kg for the lower body.

These weights will sound light to advanced athletes, so remember they are based on the average healthy person. It is always better to decide that the weights you are using are too light and be able to increase them rather than starting too heavy and hurting yourself.

Is lifting weights bad for joints, especially the knees?

In many ways the opposite is true. Strength training has a positive effect on the four structural components of all articulated joints: bones, muscles, ligaments and tendons. However if you have a pre-existing injury or condition, then loading a joint may slow down the healing process, so get the joint working well with your bodyweight first, then when it is fully healed begin to introduce light weight training.

When do I breathe?

I find that nine times out of 10 people are already breathing correctly when they ask this question. Exercise teachers say a lot of things, it seems, just for the sake of something to say and coaching breathing is one of those things. For the vast majority of the moves you would breathe out naturally during the exertion phase (hard bit). However, during a handful of the moves actually holding the breath has a positive effect on the exercise, because it creates intra-abdominal pressure (IAP), which is is a natural reaction that stabilises the torso internally. On the few moves where it is desirable to get the IAP effect, I have noted this in the notes on technique.

As a woman, I'm worried that using weights will make my muscles bigger – is that true?

Building muscle doesn't happen by accident; it requires intensive lifting of heavy weights, an increased consumption of protein and often nutritional supplements. However, females don't easily increase their muscle size because they don't have the same muscle-building hormone levels that men do, particularly of testosterone.

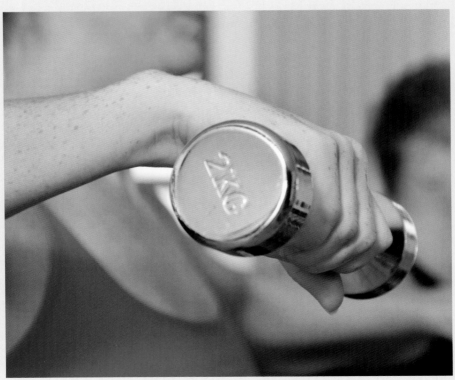

With that fear laid to rest, let's focus on the desirable outcome of lifting weights for females (and men): the potential to improve muscle tone. Muscle tone is the body's natural reaction to a muscle being worked against resistance. A toned muscle feels firm, and when it is covered by only healthy amounts of body fat, the contours of the muscle can actually be seen through the skin.

Can I lose weight by working with dumbbells?

If a reduction of fat levels is the goal, weight training is not only desirable but essential. Lifting weights is at least as effective for fat burning as cardio training and, in fact, when you take into account the 'after-burn' effects of weight training, where the body continues to burn calories following cardio and strength training activity, it is more effective. After-burn or, to use the full name, excess post-exercise oxygen consumption (EPOC) is the human body's method for erasing the oxygen debt that occurs when we undergo strenuous activity. Increased oxygen consumption occurs in conjunction with increased consumption of fuel, which is taken from subcutaneous fat stores. If this phenomenon is new to you, the chances are you have heard it previously referred to as 'speeding up your metabolism'. However, this process isn't speeding up your metabolism in the truest sense, as this really occurs when you increase lean muscle mass (tone). But, since you gain muscle tone through resistance training, when you combine the two physical adaptations you get a higher consumption of energy (and therefore fat loss) in a person who is physically active compared to a sedentary individual.

Will dumbbell training give me better muscle definition?

The short answer is yes. But the individual results will depend upon the frequency and intensity of the lifting and the overall visual effect is highly dependent upon your body fat percentage (the total weight of your body fat divided by your total weight). To have a lean defined appearance males require a body fat percentage of approximately 5–10 per cent and females 10–15 per cent. These figures will sound high to those interested in the ultra lean or 'ripped' appearance you see on competitive body builders, but it is important to understand that pre-competition bodybuilders undergo an extreme regime to eradicate the fluid and fat in their bodies. This is an obsessive approach to diet and exercise and is, therefore, physically and practically unsustainable for long periods of time.

For the average person lifting weights is the most practical way of developing muscle definition, and as long as the diet is sensible and contains enough protein, the amount of muscle definition you achieve will correspond with the frequency and intensity of your training.

Should I wear a weight lifting belt?

No. Weight lifting belts are part of the 'old school' method and belong to the era before we recognised the importance of core strength. Weights belts have a role in power lifting competitions and during some maximum weight lifts. However, rather than protect your back, wearing a belt makes it weaker over time because you become dependent on the support it gives and, thus, don't build up your stabilising muscles.

Is it good to carry dumbbells when I walk, jog or run?

No. For weights to have any effect on the intensity of your workout they need to be heavier than the tiny 1kg weights people often walk with. If you carry heavy weights when walking or jogging it will have a negative effect upon your walking or running gait. This is because having the weights in your hands at the ends of your limbs significantly affects your smooth forward propulsion. A more productive product that won't interfere with your biomechanics is a weighted vest. This adds to the weight on your muscles, but keeps the load close to your natural centre of gravity.

In some of the moves the knees joints bend past 90 degrees – is that safe?

Yes. Our knees naturally bend past 90 degrees and sitting in a squat position is a common position for many people around the world to take up without a second thought. If this is something you are not used to doing, then condition yourself to do this bending without any weights before adding any load.

What is the difference between a dumbbell and a kettlebell?

Dumbbells have their weight distributed equally between the two ends of the handles whereas on a kettlebell the weight is positioned away from the handle. This gives the effect that when a kettlebell is swung or moved quickly, the resulting inertia causes it to feel heavier than a dumbbell of equal weight.

What is the best time of the day to exercise?

The answer to this question is very subjective. If you are an athlete training almost every day, perhaps twice a day, then I would say that strength training in the morning could be more productive than at other times due to higher levels of desirable hormones being present in the bloodstream after a good nights sleep. However, in the case of a casual exerciser with an average diet, a job and busy lifestyle my answer would be to exercise at any time of the day, particularly as exercise is such a fantastic use of your valuable free time.

find your starting point

Before starting any exercise programme, test your body against the fitness/function checklist: mobility, flexibility, muscle recruitment and strength.

Before you think about picking up any weights you need to establish what your starting point is in terms of mobility, flexibility and strength. Every first consultation with a new personal training client revolves around the wish list of goals they hope to achieve. This list inevitably combines realistic goals with entirely unrealistic aims. Invariably people focus on their 'wants' rather than their 'needs' when goal setting, and there is a big difference between the two mindsets. While 'wanting' could be considered a positive attitude, it will never overcome the need to slowly expose the body to processes that will change its characteristics and ability. Men in particular want to grab the weights and start lifting, but it makes no sense to overload a muscle if you haven't given your starting point any consideration.

realistic goal setting
Want (v) 'A desired outcome'
Need (n) 'Circumstances requiring some course of action'

By identifying your needs, your goals may not sound so spectacular but you are more likely to achieve better and longer term results, and your progress through the fitness process will be considerably more productive. Therefore, rather than thinking about the ultimate outcome, think instead of resolutions to the 'issues'.

fitness/function checklist
The checklist you need to put your body through before making a grab for the heaviest dumbbell is very simple and logical. Our ability to lift weights relies on a combination of:

- Mobility
- Flexibility
- Muscle recruitment
- Strength

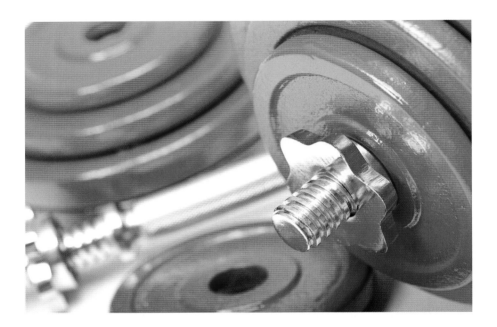

If any of these vital components is neglected, it will have a knock-on effect on your progress. For example, while you may have the raw strength in your quadriceps to squat with a heavy weight, if you do not have a full range of motion in the ankle joints and sufficient flexibility in the calf muscles, then your squat will inevitably be of poor quality. Likewise, in gyms it is common to see men who have overtrained their chest muscles to such an extent that they can no longer achieve scapular retraction (they are round shouldered and therefore demonstrate poor technique in moves that require them to raise their arms above their heads).

This type of checklist is traditionally the most overlooked component of strength training and, while testing weight, body fat levels and cardiac performance is now a regular occurrence in the fitness industry, the introduction of screening for quality of movement has taken a much longer time to become a priority. This, despite a self-administered assessment being as simple as looking in the mirror.

assess, don't guess

If you want results from any type of physical exercise then starting a programme without first assessing your ability and quality of movement is like going on an unfamiliar journey without first looking at a map – you might reach your destination but you also might get lost. This section of the book aims to help you think about human movement and the way it relates to strength and conditioning training.

There is no better summary of how important mobility is than in one of my favourite sayings: 'Use it or lose it'. What does this mean you ask? Well, I can honestly say that the one time in my life that I was at my fittest was also the time that I applied the least amount of science to my training – I simply did the things that felt good: stretching muscles, lifting weights, running fast and slow and being involved in lots of sports that combined speed, balance and coordination – basically I was as active as you could imagine a person could be. Throughout this time I can't remember being injured or suffering any aches or pains – I put this down to the fact that unlike most people I didn't have to stand still or sit at a desk or drive a vehicle for long periods of time and therefore I didn't have any of the problems that many people seem to live with these days – I was so active that all the imbalances, aches and pains that start to occur when you become sedentary were kept at bay, so what I am saying with my statement of 'use it or lose it' is simple, if your body exists in a perfect 'bubble' of activity and recovery then you are most likely to be strong, mobile and flexible but as soon as you start to not use your body for productive physical tasks then you start to lose the luxury of being able to do so without a second thought.

Today, the assessment of 'functional movement', or biomechanical screening, is its own specialised industry within the world of fitness. Those working in orthopaedics and conventional medical rehabilitation have always followed some form of standardised assessment where they test the function of the nerves, muscles and bones before forming an opinion of a patient's condition. Becoming a trained practitioner takes many years of study and practice. Not only must a practitioner gain knowledge of a wide spectrum of potential conditions, but just as importantly they must understand when and how to treat their patient, or when they need to refer them to other colleagues in the medical profession. Having been subjected to and taught many different approaches to movement screening, in my mind, the challenge isn't establishing there is something 'wrong', rather it is *knowing* what to do to rectify the issue.

mobility and flexibility

The most common problem limiting quality of movement in the average person is a lack of mobility and flexibility, which can be provisionally tested using the standing twist and the overhead squat assessment (see below).

To understand why mobility is key to human movement, think how as babies we start to move independently. We are born with mobility and flexibility, then we progressively develop stability, balance and then increasing amounts of strength. As we get older we may experience injuries, periods of inactivity and, to some extent, stress which all contribute towards a progressive reduction of mobility. There is no better summary of how important mobility is than in one of my favourite sayings: 'Use it or lose it'. If you sit for extended periods or fail to move through the three planes of motion (see page 151), then you invariably become restricted in your motion. With this in mind, I hope you can see that lifting weights without first addressing mobility issues is like trying to build the walls of a house before you have completed the foundations.

The following two mobility tests challenge the entire length of the kinetic chain (the actions and reaction to force that occur throughout the bones, muscles and nerves whenever dynamic motion or force is required from the body) and help to reveal if you are ready to move beyond bodyweight moves to begin adding the additional load of dumbbells. This test focuses on the following key areas of the shoulders, the mid-thoracic spine, the pelvis, the knees, ankles and feet. Any limitation of mobility, flexibility or strength in these areas will show up as either an inability to move smoothly through the exercise or an inability to hold the body in the desired position.

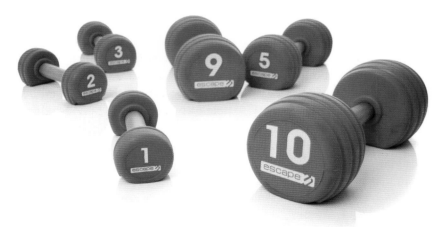

Test 1 standing twist

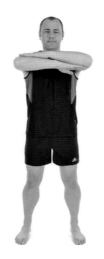 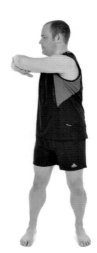

This is the less dramatic of the two mobility tests and serves to highlight if you have any pain that only presents when you move through the outer regions of your range of movement, and also if you have a similar range of motion between rotations on the left and right sides of your body.

● Stand with your feet beneath your hips.
● Raise your arms to chest height then rotate as far as you can to the right, noting how far you can twist.
● Repeat the movement to the left.
● Perform the movement slowly so that no 'extra twist' is achieved using speed and momentum.

Your observation is trying to identify any pain and/or restriction of movement. If you find either, it might be the case that this reduces after a warm-up or a few additional repetitions of this particular movement. If you continue to experience pain, you should consider having it assessed by a physiotherapist or sports therapist.

Test 2 overhead squat (OHS)

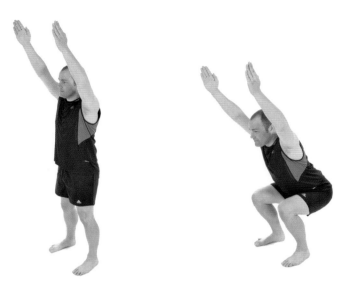

I've used the OHS test over 5000 times as part of my S.A.F.E. approach to exercise and I have found it to be the quickest and easiest way of looking at basic joint and muscle function without getting drawn in to speculative diagnosis of what is and isn't working properly. If you can perform this move without any pain or restriction, then you will find most of the moves in this book achievable. There is no pass or fail, rather you will fall into one of two categories: 'Good' or 'could do better'. If you cannot achieve any of the key requirements of the OHS move, then it is your body's way of flagging up that you are tight and/or weak in that particular area. This, in turn, could mean you have an imbalance, pain or an untreated injury, which may not prevent you from exercising, but you should probably get checked out by a physiotherapist or sports therapist.

Perform this exercise barefoot and in front of a full-length mirror so that you can gain maximum information from the observation of your whole body. See table 1 for a list of key body regions to observe during this test. (This move also doubles up as a brilliant warm-up for lifting weights.)

- Stand with feet pointing straight ahead and at hip width.
- Have your hands in the 'thumbs-up position' and raise your arms above your head, keeping them straight, into the top of a 'Y' position (with your body being the bottom of the 'Y'). Your arms are in the correct position when they are back far enough to disappear from your peripheral vision.

- The squat down is slow and deep, so take a slow count of six to get down by bending your knees. The reason we go slow is so you do not allow gravity to take over and merely slump down. Also, by going slow you get a chance to see and feel how everything is moving through the six key areas.

The magic of this move is that you will be able to see and feel where your problem spots are and, even better, the test becomes the solution, as simply performing it regularly helps with your quality of movement. Stretch out any area that feels tight and aim to work any area that feels weak.

Table 1 Key body regions to observe in the overhead squat

Body region	Good position	Bad position
Neck		
Shoulders		
Mid-thoracic spine		
Hips		

Knees			
Ankles and feet			

As you perform the OHS you are looking for control and symmetry throughout and certain key indicators that all is well:

- Neck: you keep good control over your head movements and are able to maintain the arm lift without pain in the neck.
- Shoulders: in the start position and throughout the move you are aiming to have both arms lifted above the head and retracted enough so that they are outside your peripheral vision (especially when you are in the deep part of the squat). In addition to observing the shoulders look up at your arms to the hands – throughout the OHS you should aim to have your thumbs pointing behind you.
- Mid-thoracic spine: there is no instruction to keep your back straight, so in this area of the body you are looking for 'flow' rather than clunking movements.
- Hips: imagine a straight line drawn directly down the centre of your body. Around the hips you are looking to see if you shift your weight habitually to one side, rather than keeping it evenly spread between both sides.
- Knees: the most common observation is the knees touching during the OHS, suggesting a weakness in the glutes. Less common is the knees parting, showing weakness in the inner thigh. Good technique is when your knees move forwards as you bend the legs. Note that clicking and crunching noises don't always suggest a problem unless they are accompanied by pain.
- Ankles and feet: the most obvious issue is the heels lifting from the floor, suggesting short achilles and calf muscles. Less obvious are the flattening of the foot arches that cause the feet to roll inward (overpronation) or the foot rolling outward (underpronation). Ideally, the foot should be in a neutral position.

If when you do the OHS in front of the mirror you observe any of the visual signals that suggest you don't have optimal movement qualities it really isn't the end of the world, in fact, most people find that they are tight in some areas (if not all of them) when they first try this test. The absolutely fantastic news is that if you do spot any issues, performing the OHS as an exercise, rather than merely a test, will improve your movement pattern, joint range and muscle actions over time.

overhead squat: the results

My rule is that if you cannot perform a perfect OHS, with none of the key warning signs listed above, then you are not ready to perform the power moves in the exercise portfolio. So, use the OHS as a guide to whether your body is as ready as your mind is to start doing the toughest, most challenging, exercises. If you find by doing the OHS that your body is not ready, don't think of it as a setback, but rather as a blessing: you are following a training method that is in tune with how the body works rather than one that merely sets out to punish it.

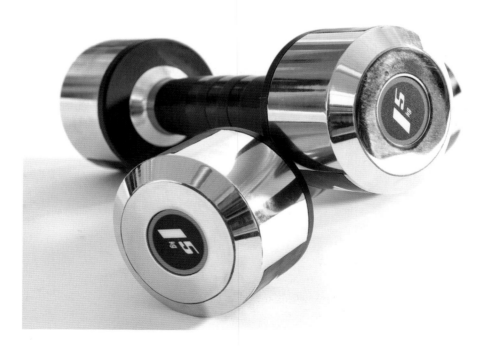

isolation vs integration

While intensity can be great, when you isolate your muscles you do not get the highly beneficial activity created by the rest of the kinetic chain. I am certainly not saying isolation moves are not productive, but with the biggest obstacle to exercise being a lack of time, integration work is going to have an instant usable impact on the entire body.

All movements that we do in training or everyday life can be classified as either isolation or integration moves. The vast majority of isolation moves have been created/invented to work specific muscles on their own, with the primary intention of fatiguing that muscle by working it in isolation, usually moving only one joint of the skeleton. Integration, or compound, moves are less of an invention and more of an adaptation of movement patterns that we perform in everyday life. They are designed to work groups of muscles across multiple joints all at the same time.

In real life we never isolate. Even when only a few joints are moving there is a massive number of muscles bracing throughout the body to let the prime muscles do their job. As you go about an average day I doubt you give a second thought to how you are moving. If you take the time to watch the world go by for a few hours you will notice that human movement consists of just a few combinations of movements that together create the millions of potential moves we (hopefully) achieve everyday. Everything, and I mean everything, we do boils down to the following key movements:

- Push
- Pull
- Twist
- Squat
- Lunge
- Bend
- Walk
- Run
- Jump

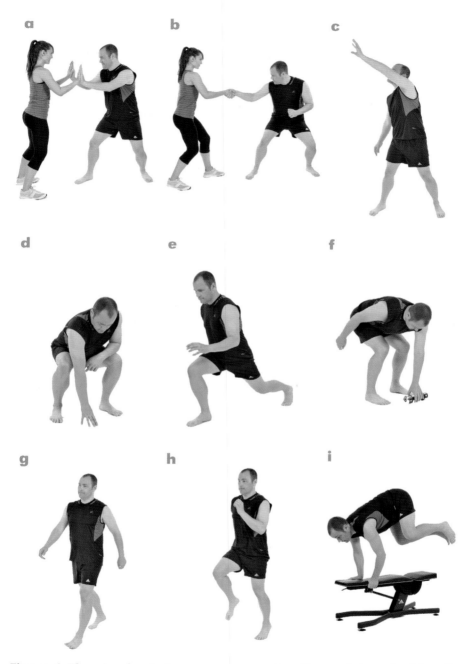

Figure 1 The nine basic human movement patterns: (a) push, (b) pull, (c) twist, (d) squat, (e) lunge, (f) bend, (g) walk, (h) run and (i) jump

All of these movements are integrated. I am certainly not the first person to make this observation, but it constantly amazes me how my industry manages to complicate exercise. With this observation in mind, I am not a huge fan of old fashioned machines that isolate small areas of muscle to work them apparently more intensely. While intensity can be great, when you isolate you do not get the highly beneficial activity created by the rest of the kinetic chain. I am certainly not saying isolation moves are not productive, but with the biggest obstacle to exercise being a lack of time, integration work is going to have an instant usable impact on the entire body.

Because of this, I moved away from using exercises that focused on isolation many years ago. When I first started using twisting and bending moves in training, those who used weights machines with seats, and even seatbelts, to fix them into position suggested that it looked dangerous. However, in reality I was lifting weight in such a way that the moves could be directly compared to how I moved in my chosen sports of athletics and rugby – my sprint start required me to explode out of the starting blocks, driving through one leg at a time, and in rugby I needed to be conditioned to push, pull and twist all of the time. Therefore, exercises such as lunges, cross chops and single-leg squats were all perfect for this, but they were far from mainstream exercises.

That was many years ago, and since then a completely new section of the fitness industry has sprung up that specialises in what we now call functional, or core, training. Of course, I'm not claiming to have invented this approach to exercise; in fact, that honour must go to a guy back in Ancient Roman times, who decided one day to start swinging a weight around: these days we would call it a kettlebell.

Because of these conclusions, I find it increasingly difficult to justify performing only isolation exercises myself and with my clients, and multiple muscle integration moves are at the heart of all of my training programmes. Subsequently, the majority of the moves in this book are integrated, designed to achieve maximum results in the most economical amount of time.

learn it, then work it

As we have discovered, you must walk before you can run in any exercise method, and the body works best if you learn the activity prior to engaging in exercise, so that you will positively soak up the benefits.

Lifting weights is very natural with hardly any complex skills required to achieve results. However, that is not to say you cannot do it incorrectly. In fact, along with failed runners, re-building the confidence of people who have tried weight training and then failed or injured themselves has featured frequently in my working life. Because of this, I use the phrase 'learn it, then work it' to encourage people to take time to 'imprint' good quality movement patterns upon their bodies.

how to 'learn it, then work it'

How do you know what 'good quality' moves look like? Simply put, the move should look smooth and controlled and should not create pain in your joints. Aim to perform the concentric and eccentric phases (the lift and lower phases) at the same speed – lift for two counts and lower for two counts. When power and speed becomes more of an objective for you, aim to lift for one count and lower for two counts.

You can perform moves at slower speeds, but that then moves away from how we move/function in day to day life, rarely do we do any movement in slow motion just for the sake of it. It is really only beneficial to perform slow or super slow (quarter-speed) moves if you are training for specific sport activities, so as to prolong the time each muscle is under tension (known as 'time under tension'). Therefore, move at a natural speed: athletes and sports people train at 'real time' once they have learned the required movement pattern, so without even knowing it they are 'learning it, then working it'.

The beauty of grounding your workout in the 'learn it, then work it' approach is that by keeping the approach simple, achievable and functional you won't get tied up with methods that either do not work, or have ridiculous expectations of how much time you are going to dedicate to your fitness regime. It is quite often that I see people in gyms who perform difficult versions of exercises that are clearly beyond their level of ability – presuming because they think difficult/ advance must equal quicker results. The obvious signs are that they can't control the weights or their body seems overpowered by the movements it is being asked to do – learn it, then work it relates to most physical tasks in life but especially sport. For example, if you have tennis lessons the first thing you would learn would be to make contact with the ball slowly rather than starting with the fastest hardest movements. So the key is to simply switch off your instincts to 'work hard' until you are satisfied that you can move correctly by maintaining quality and control throughout all the repetitions.

As you get more adventurous and diverse with your exercise remember all your goals are achievable: remember, if you're moving you're improving.

'learn it, then work it' in sport

Practising movements in weight training is paralleled in all performance-based sports. Athletes routinely perform low intensity 'drills', which echo the moves they need to make in their sport. For example, during almost every track session, sprinters practise knee lifts, heel flicks and other bounding exercises to improve their quality of movement and condition their muscles in a highly functional manner.

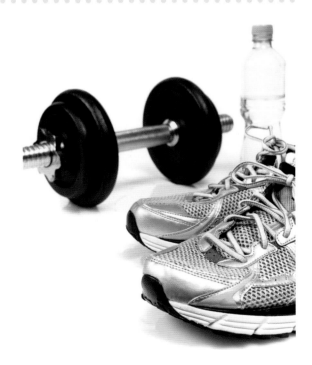

first you need stability

Stability is the first key ingredient to ensuring safe and effective exercise, the basic building block to everything that follows in this book.

To perform exercise safely and effectively, we have to firstly ensure our body is stable. The essence of stability is the ability to control and transfer force throughout the body. All human movement is, in fact, a chain of events involving the brain, the nervous system, muscles, fascia, ligaments and tendons. So, while a simple move like a bicep curl may appear to involve only activity from the shoulder down to the hand, in reality there is a chain of events that occur to ensure that the right amount of force is applied and that the two ends of the bicep are tethered to a stable base.

In essence, wherever there is visible movement in the body, there are always invisible reactions occurring within the kinetic chain to facilitate this movement.

The engine room of all this activity is in the deep muscles of the trunk and involves the:

- Transversus abdominus (TA)
- Multifidi (MF)
- Internal obliques
- Five layers of muscle and fascia that make up the pelvic floor.

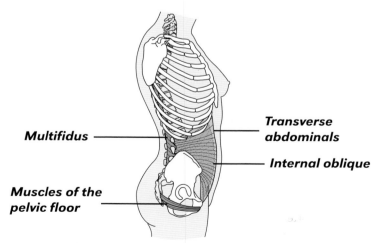

Figure 2 The deep muscles of the trunk are crucial for stability

These muscles work as a team and their simultaneous contraction is known as 'co-contraction'. This complex muscle activity produces intra-abdominal pressure (IAP) and it is the creation of this pressure that stabilises the lumber spine. The misconception that the transversus abdominus looks like a 'belt' around the torso no doubt led fitness instructors to continuously advise clients to pull their stomach in (hollow the abdominal muscles), thinking that this would amplify the stability of the spine. However, it is not simply the recruitment of these muscles that instills strength and stability, but, more importantly, when they are recruited. In effect, they should have been advising clients to 'switch on' (brace their core).

remember: don't hollow your abs

Pulling in, or hollowing, the abs actually makes you less able to stabilise. If you imagine a tree that is perfectly vertical, but then you chop in or hollow out one side, the structure of the tree becomes less stable. I have two ways of coaching the correct technique to avoid hollowing the abs, depending on the client:

1 Switch on your abs as if you were going to get punched in the stomach, or
2 Engage the abs in the same way as if were about to be tickled.

Both methods achieve the desired outcome – with only a few of my male clients actually insisting that I really do hit them!

Stability is, therefore, a goal in everything that we do. However, we shouldn't have to undertake yet more training just to achieve core stability, rather we should ensure that the everyday movements we make encourage the muscles deep inside the trunk to work correctly during dynamic movements, and that the stabilisation is instinctive, as opposed to something that we have to remind ourselves to do every time. For instance, if you drop an egg in the kitchen and very quickly squat and make a grab to catch it, you don't stop to think: 'Did I line up my feet, pull my stomach in and keep my head up?' Actually, your body will have fired off a co-contraction which enabled you to grab the egg before it hit the ground (or, at least, make a good attempt). When I use this analogy to explain the concept of stability to my clients, they often get a twinkle in their eye, for if this process is instinctive, why should they continue to train? The reality, however, if that you still have to exercise that inclination to keep the system working properly: 'use it, or lose it'.

In the workout sessions later in this book, you will find that almost all the moves are classified as being good for stability. Since stability is the first stage of development, you might assume the strength and power moves that follow are more productive because they are more 'intense'. While this is true, that intensity will only be constructive if the body has the ability to control and direct all that extra force, which can only be learned through the stability moves.

the development of core stability in the fitness industry

During the 1990s, there were only three components of fitness that personal trainers focused on with the average client (by 'average' I mean a person looking for fitness gains rather than to compete in sport). Cardio was the route to cardiovascular efficiency and was the most obvious tool for weight loss; strength training isolated the larger muscle groups and gymnasiums were filled with straight line machines; and we only worked on flexibility because we knew we had to, but the chosen method was predominately the least productive type of stretching, i.e. static.

Then, it seems almost from nowhere, there was a new ingredient to every workout: core stability. New equipment such as Swiss balls and modern versions of wobble boards, such as the Reebok Core Board® and the BOSU® (Both sides up), increased the wave of enthusiasm for this type of training as, of course, did the new popularity for the more physical versions of yoga and Pilates.

In retrospect, we in the fitness industry could have thought to ourselves that we had been doing everything wrong up to that point. However, the reality is that rather than being 'wrong' we were just learning as we went along. In fact, many of the methods that suddenly became mainstream had been used in sports training for years before, but without the 'label' of core stability, and rather than treating them as an individual component, we trained them instinctively as part of our dynamic strength moves using body weight or free weights.

add some strength

The second key ingredient, there are several types of strength that you can gain performing these exercises with dumbbells.

When trying to establish a client's fitness objectives, 'I want to improve my strength' is often the only information given to a personal trainer. This seemingly simple request requires much more detail if you are going to achieve the outcome that is really desired.

The one-line definition of strength could be summed up as: An ability to exert a physical force against resistance. However, this catch-all is not specific enough when you are dealing with strength. In fact, there are three main types of strength:

1 Strength endurance: achieved when you aim to exert force many times in close succession.
2 Elastic strength: achieved when you make fast contractions to regain a position or posture.
3 Maximum strength: our ability over a single repetition to generate our greatest amount of force.

Each of these specific types of strength can be achieved using dumbbells either as individual components or preferably as part of an integrated approach.

Unless you are an athlete training for an event that requires a disproportionate amount of either endurance, elastic or maximum strength, then the integration of functional training methods will create a body that is more designed to cope with day to day life and amateur sports. While strength is an adaptation that the body willingly accepts, the reality is that changes take time, so treat strength gains as something that happens over weeks, months and years rather than mere days.

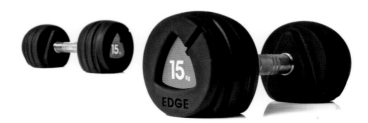

power beats size

The development of power, rather than size, in muscles is not only a more rapid process, but is also considerably more practical, usable and functional for those men and women who have reached a point in their training where they have no need to be any 'stronger', but they want to make more of the strength they have.

Increasing the size of a muscle is a long process that requires focused attention to training and nutrition. The majority of super-huge bodybuilders need to train for hours every day and consume massive volumes of food and supplements to increase their muscle size, and this type of training often becomes an obsession – if not an addiction.

For many years people believed that training with weights and getting bigger muscles were mutually exclusive. And while body building has a cult following around the world, the reality is that training purely in the pursuit of increasing muscle size is a niche market. It is true that clients (predominately men) ask to increase the size of their muscles, but with closer scrutiny, they want to achieve an athletic physique rather than massive bulk.

Power is the ability to exert an explosive burst of movement. In everyday life it presents as bounding up stairs three at a time or pushing a heavy weight above your head. The development of power, rather than size, in muscles is not only a more rapid process, but is also considerably more practical, usable and functional for those men and women who have reached a point in their training where they have no need to be any 'stronger', but they want to make more of the strength they have.

When you get to the training stage, you will see that the power moves are, in fact, progressions of the skills that you will have already developed during your stability and strength sessions, only performed at speed. In this respect, it becomes easier to understand why I advise not to skip a stage when learning movement patterns.

power and agility

Think of power as a very close relation of agility; you don't learn agility by overloading and working while fatigued, rather you develop it by achieving quality over quantity. In fact, introducing yourself to the pursuit of power can mean performing the moves without any weights and simply performing the movements fast, as athletic power is actually a finely tuned combination of speed and strength.

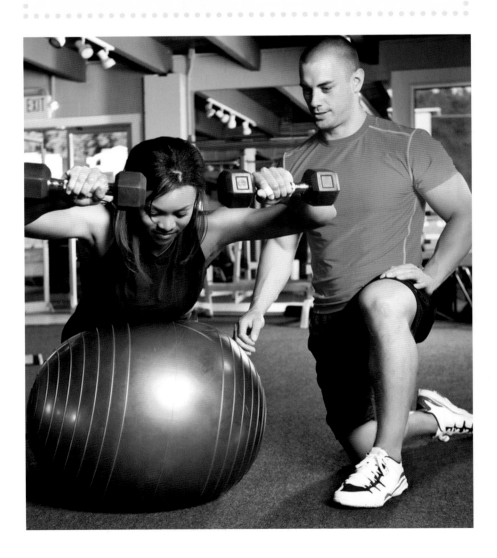

2 the portfolio of moves

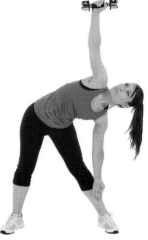

which moves should I do?

This section contains a portfolio of moves that I have selected from those I use every day with my personal training clients and are based on the principles I explained in the first part of this book. The only moves that have made it into this book are those that deserve to be here – every one of these moves is tried and tested to ensure it gets results, in fact, I have spent hundreds of hours using them myself and thousands of hours teaching them to my personal training clients, who over the years have included men and women from 16 to 86 years old, from size zero through to 280lbs. These clients have, justifiably, only been interested in the moves that work – and that is what you have here in this portfolio.

It is not an exhaustive list of moves, simply because many extra moves that could have been included are really just subtle adaptations of those included here. For instance, changes to foot position and the amount of bend that you have in your arms and legs will encourage the body to recruit slightly different muscles, but I would class these as adaptations rather than unique moves.

dangerous dumbbell moves

There will always be those people who dream up dumbbell moves that are dangerous, pointless or just plain stupid. A pair of dumbbells in sensible hands is a very safe product but, having spent thousands of hours in gyms all around the world, I know that there are plenty of people who think that just because they have invented an 'exercise', it must be doing 'something good' to the body.

Without even acknowledging the really crazy stuff I have seen, I simply cannot condone or include any moves that use a dumbbell in ways that were never intended. Dumbbells are not designed to be thrown or caught and, unlike a kettlebell, they are not intended to be swung between the legs. I would also recommend that you don't attempt any exercises where you swap the dumbbell between your hands mid-exercise.

presentation of the moves

I wanted to show the moves as a complete portfolio, rather than simply wrapping them up into workouts, because you are then able to see how the stability, strength and power versions relate to each other. Understanding these progressions is something I encourage of my clients because they need to know that subtle changes can make all the difference between a good use of time and a waste of it. By thinking this way you can very quickly learn all the moves because, in the majority of cases, the main movement pattern stays the same throughout the stability, strength and power progressions, with only a slight change to the length of levers (arm/foot positions), range of motion or the speed.

The third part of this book then goes on to present a selection of training sessions, designed for a range of levels, and following my method of progressing through stability, strength and power exercises. I have also provided you with a post-workout stretch session suitable for weight lifting training (see pages 121–123). Please remember that you should always warm-up before embarking on any type of exercise.

I have written the descriptions as if I am talking to you as a client – the key information for each explanation includes:

● the correct body position at the start and finish of the move;
● the movement that you are looking to create.

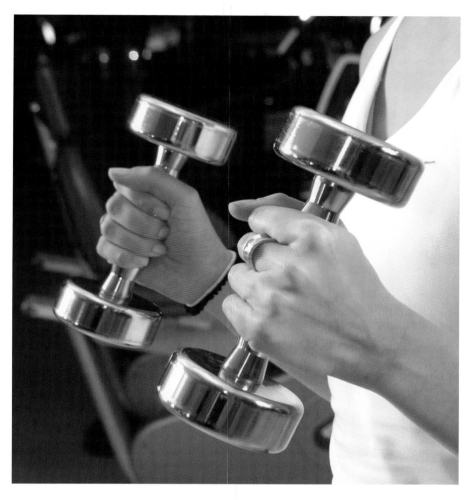

When I work with my PT clients I avoid over-coaching the movement as my goal is to see them move in a lovely 'fluid' way, where the whole movement blends together.

every muscle plays a part
I purposefully haven't included diagrams of the muscles that are targeted by each move as hopefully by now you understand that, used correctly, every muscle plays a role in every move.

reps

This is a 'learn it' section rather than 'work it'. Therefore, for the vast majority of the moves I don't talk about how many repetitions you should do of each – that information is included in the workout section in the third part of the book. How many repetitions you perform should relate to your objectives; almost all the moves can be used to improve stability, strength and power (at the same time), and the speed and resistance at which you perform it will dictate the outcome. For example, a slow squat performed with a light weight will provide stability benefits. Exactly the same move performed with a heavier weight will increase strength and the same move at speed will develop power.

weight

As speed and resistance are both subjective (one person's 'light' is another person's 'heavy'), it is simply not possible, without being in the same room as you and looking at how you move and your physical characteristics, to suggest the exact weight you should use. When you are learning the moves from this portfolio, you should use a weight that allows you to perform six to eight excellent quality repetitions. When you reach the workout sessions in the third part of the book each of the moves has a specific repetition number applied to it so that they work in context with the suggested time for each workout, i.e. 15, 30 or 45 minutes.

tricks of the trade

For each exercise, I have included a 'tricks of the trade' box which contains a nugget of information that I use to help my clients get the most out of each exercise.

key to exercises

As you move through the exercises, you will notice that each is identified by the following key words. A quick glance will tell you which element the move focuses on, what type of move it is and whether you need any additional equipment to perform it.

stability

As has been discussed earlier in the book, you don't have to use gym balls and wobble devices to get stability benefits. Stability is, essentially, a reaction within the kinetic chain in which the body says to itself: 'Switch on the muscles around the lumbo pelvic region, because this movement is looking for an anchor point to latch on to'. On this basis, you don't improve stability when you are sat down, neither do you generally improve it when a move involves just one joint.

strength

We could get all deep and meaningful about biomechanics here, but to qualify as a strength move, the exercise needs to be making you move a force through space using muscle contractions. Therefore anything that only involves momentum is a waste of time because you are just going along for the ride and not actively contracting your muscles. However, don't confuse speed with momentum – speed is good, especially when mixed with strength, because that combination develops the highly desirable power.

power

Every time you read the word 'power' you need to think of speed, and vice versa. The maths and physics required to understand how we measure power are enough to make you glaze over, and in reality you are much better off measuring your power ability by doing a simple time-trial sprint, or time yourself over a set number of repetitions, rather than trying to calculate exactly how much power you are exerting for a specific exercise.

If you want more power, you need to move fast, but you need to be able to maintain speed while pushing or pulling a weight (that weight could be an object or your own body). For example, you might have a guy who can skip across a shot put circle faster than the other guy when not holding and throwing the shot, but he is only speedy. The guy who can move fast and launch the shot (using strength) is the one with all the power.

isolation

This is a move where you are intentionally using only one muscle (or group, such as the quadriceps) to move a weight. This means that usually you are also only moving one joint. There is nothing wrong with isolation moves and they are particularly good at forcing several muscles in the body to grow (for example, the biceps, triceps and quadriceps). However, they need to be part of an organised approach to strength training, because if you only do isolation moves you won't develop good movement patterns. Think of it this way: if you were a tree, there would be no point having really strong branches without a trunk and root system. Isolation training, without incorporating integration moves, develops strength that you will find hard to use for anything other than more isolation moves.

integration/compound

This is a move that will have a beneficial knock-on effect on every physical task or sporting challenge you undertake. Integration moves can usually be classed as being beneficial for the core muscles. They might also be referred to as 'functional' moves (however, this is an overused term, as some people say that swinging a kettlebell is 'functional', but I can't think of any activity in everyday life where I swing a weight between my legs rather than over my head). Integration is essentially moving the dumbbell using multiple muscles, ranges of motion and joints. You may have guessed by now that I'm a big fan of this set of moves – why bother working muscles one at a time when you can train them to work as a team and get more done in less time?

don't waste your time

Moves which include the above 'trash' symbol, fall into two groups; those that actually achieve nothing, usually because gravity or momentum is creating all the movement rather than a muscle contraction, and those that give you the impression that you are doing good because they are causing fatigue (pain) in muscles. However, what you may not have realised is that the pain you are feeling actually comes from a tiny postural muscle like for example teres minor that you have suddenly loaded in a way unsympathetic to the way it functions best.

bench

These moves require a bench to perform them. Ensure that the bench you use is specifically designed for weight training. Most training benches adjust so that they can be used flat or at an incline of 30, 45 and 70 degrees. For exercises that require only a flat surface, a fitness step can be used as a platform to lie on, but do not adapt them to incline. The Reebok® Deck offers an excellent solution for home use as it provides all the features of a fitness step as well as adjusting to 30, 45 and 70 degree inclines.

ball

These moves require a ball to perform them. In the world of fitness there are good balls and there are bad balls; make sure that the ball you are using has load capacity strong enough to hold you and the weight of the dumbbells. (See *The Total Gym Ball Workout* (Bloomsbury, 2011) by this author for everything you could ever wish to know about gym ball exercises).

the classic moves

These are without doubt the need-to-know dumbbell moves. With a few exceptions, the oldest and most popular dumbbell moves are also the most effective. Long before the term 'core' came along athletes and bodybuilders were practising the basic moves that work the prime movers in our body, which in turn developed integrated strength. Isolation moves emerged when people became more interested in the cosmetic effects of weight training rather than the performance-enhancing effects.

Sadly, it seems an entire generation of personal trainers missed out on learning these classic moves because weight machines became the dominant force in most gymnasiums. Fitness machines have since significantly improved, but if you want to develop a great foundation in the skill of lifting weights that will help you to keep fit and strong throughout your entire active adult life, then these are the moves that you need to perfect.

As a self-confessed trend watcher and trend predictor in the fitness industry I am pleased to say that I have seen a real increase in the number of people in gyms who are using these classic free weight exercises on a regular basis. Classic is a term that should only be bestowed upon something that has managed to stand the test of time. All of the classic moves and the best of the best moves in this portfolio have earned their place in this portfolio as a result of thousands of hours training and coaching, and I predict they will still be worthy of the title in another 40 years.

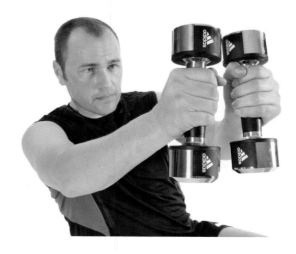

exercise 1 bicep curl, under grip

• **stability** • **strength** • **power** • **isolation**

 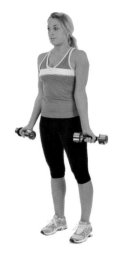

 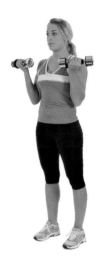

- Stand with your feet together, i.e. as wide as your pelvis or you will hit the sides of your legs with the dumbbell.
- With your palms facing forward and your upper arm hanging vertically*, lift the weight up until you have closed your elbow joint as far as it will go.
- Then, lower the dumbbell back to the start position.

* Some personal trainers tell you to keep your elbows in, to encourage you to isolate the bicep muscle, but that's not really how the body works. Personally, if a little bit of additional muscle is recruited in a move, I don't mind – and it's natural.

tricks of the trade

What can you possibly do to a bicep curl to make it more interesting? With my clients, if their attention starts to wander I make them change their foot position every couple of reps, so they shift their weight from one foot to the other and stand in a slightly split stance (one foot forward). This has no adverse effect on the curl and is also beneficial for coordination.

exercise 2 bicep reverse curl, over grip

● stability ● strength ● power ● isolation

a
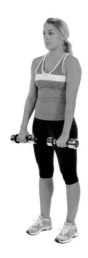

b
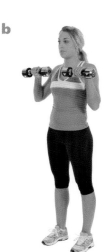

● Stand with your feet no wider than your pelvis and hold the dumbbell so that your knuckles are facing forward.
● Keep the upper arms hanging vertically, then using your biceps lift the dumbbell up until you have closed the elbow joint completely.
● Then, lower the weight back to the start position.

tricks of the trade
There is a huge temptation to lean forward during this move. When my clients cheat in this way I make them touch their butt cheeks and shoulders against a wall (touching, not leaning), and then do the the curls – you simply can't cheat.

exercise 3 bicep curl 21s

● stability ● strength ● power ● isolation

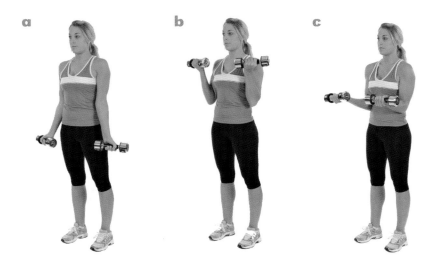

a   b   c

These are deceptively hard! The aim is to perform the three sets of seven reps immediately after each other. Why do we do this? Mainly because the biceps are very resilient muscles that do not often have to function through their full range every time they are used, so this approach is very good at creating a reaction.

● For the first seven reps, lift the dumbbell through the first half of your range of motion.
● Follow with the second set of seven reps, where you should lift the weight from halfway to the end of your range of motion.
● Finally, for the third set of seven reps lift the weight through the complete range of motion.

tricks of the trade
Whatever weight my clients think they can lift during this move, it will usually be 25 per cent less in reality. A nice personal trainer will tell you this, a nasty one will let you suffer and potentially fail the set.

exercise 4 overhead triceps press

● **stability** ● **strength** ● **power** ● **isolation**

 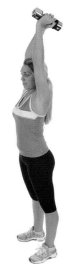 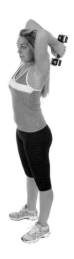

This exercise is best done in front of a mirror so you can see where the dumbbell is.

● Stand with your feet a little bit wider than pelvis width.
● Lift the dumbbell above your head and hold the shaft with both hands.
● Start at the top and lower the dumbbell behind your head, bending at the elbow.
● As soon as it touches your body push it back up to the start position.

tricks of the trade
The mirror is good because you should be able to look at yourself throughout the move. As a personal trainer, I act as the mirror and make my clients aware of when they are in the wrong position. The best solution is simply to stand in front of my clients, as this means they naturally keep their head up to maintain eye contact.

exercise 5 single-arm triceps press

• stability • strength • power • integration

a

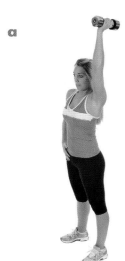

b

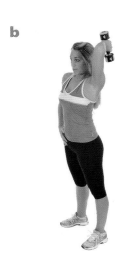

This exercise is also best done in front of a mirror so you can see where the dumbbell is. If you start with your right arm, have your right foot slightly in front of the left. The nice thing about doing one arm at a time is that you will get some work out of the pecs as well because you naturally shift your weight forward as you drive the dumbbell into the air.

● Hold the dumbbell in one hand and lift it above your head, with your arms fully extended.
● Bend your arm at the elbow and lower the dumbbell.
● Push it back up again using the triceps.

tricks of the trade
Shift your bodyweight around from foot to foot and also to the ball of the foot and heels – try it, you will find that you actually stay more focused on the arm movement than when you were standing still.

exercise 6 wrist curls, over grip

• **strength** • **power** • **isolation** • **bench**

a
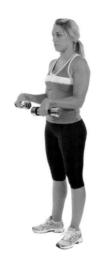

b
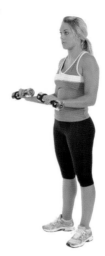

The muscles used in this movement tend to be weaker than the under grip version – if you look at your wrist this is understandable because you have more flesh on the underside than you do on the top. This exercise can also be performed standing or sitting on a bench.

- Stand up and hold your wrist in a position that allows it to move like a hinge above your knee.
- Keep your palms down and lower and lift the dumbbell.

tricks of the trade

This is the weakest range of motion for most people, so leave this move until the very end of a workout otherwise your grip will be affected for the rest of the exercises.

exercise 7 wrist curls, under grip

● strength ● power ● isolation

a

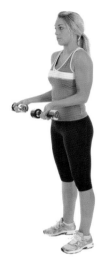

b

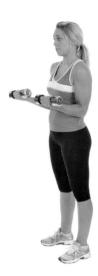

- Stand with feet apart, elbows at right angles and palms up.
- You need to remember that the range of motion here is determined by bones rather than flexibility, so don't force the joint to go further than it wants to.
- Relaxing the fingers at the end of the down phase will create work for the hand muscle as well as the wrist, but don't relax the grip too much as you are likely to drop the weight.

tricks of the trade

Despite the small amount of muscle bulk in the wrist area you will be surprised how much you can lift on this move. However, be sure to start light and progress slowly because the wrist is full of ligaments and tendons that take longer to condition than the blood-rich muscle tissue.

exercise 8 dead lift

• stability • strength • power • integration

a
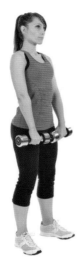

b
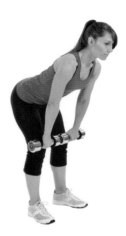

My mantra 'learn it, then work it' is key here, so practise this movement without any weights before you add extra load to your muscles and joints.

- Stand with your feet as wide apart as your armpits.
- Let the weights just hang in front of you then lower them towards the floor (that's the easy part because gravity is in charge).
- When your hamstrings reach the point that they want to stop you going any lower, stand up.
- Watch the line that the dumbbells go through – they should be going straight down and straight up again, any swing forward or back suggests the weight is too light or that you have a tight spot somewhere in your hamstrings or glutes.

tricks of the trade

The smart people practise the dead lift without a weight so that they almost pre-programme the move into their muscles and brain. An excellent practice tool is a wooden pole, because if the pole hits your knees you are too stiff or unstable to do this move with heavy weights.

53

exercise 9 deltoid raise front

• stability • strength • power • integration

a
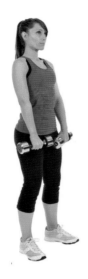

b
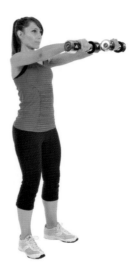

Just to clear one thing up here. When we work the deltoids we don't isolate the anterior, middle or posterior section of the muscle. Each of the sections works all of the time, but depending upon the movement each section will take on variable amounts of the load.

- Except for when using really heavy weights on this exercise, stand with you feet in whatever position is most comfortable, which means either with your feet hip width apart or in a split stance (one foot forward). If you are braving a very heavy dumbbell then a wide stance will be better.
- Before you start the lift you **must** retract your scapular (in other words, pull your shoulders back) otherwise your deltoids (one of the shoulder muscles) can't function as well as they should.
- Lift the dumbbell up to chin height. Any higher and you will again be asking the slightly isolated anterior deltoid to move in a way that it isn't designed to. I find that lifting slightly off centre is kinder on the shoulder joint than lifting straight up in front.
- And please, lower the weight under control – the eccentric phase is more than half the reason for doing this move.

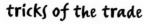

tricks of the trade

This exercise needs to flow. In the past you would have been coached to keep the rest of the body very still as you lifted the weight up, but I encourage my clients to think about and feel the muscle activity that is occurring through the upper back and all the way down to the buttocks.

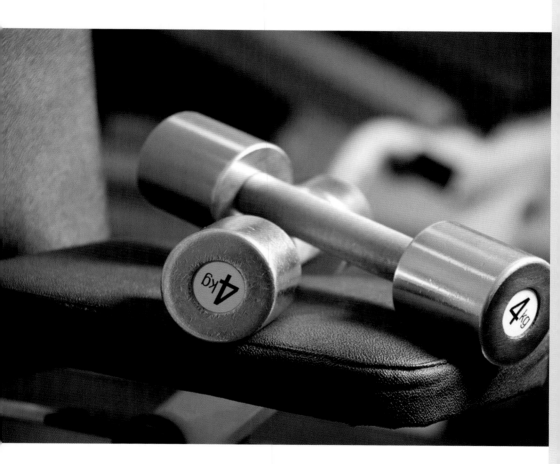

exercise 10 deltoid raise side

• stability • strength • power • integration

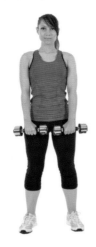

a

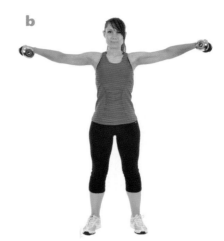

b

- Stand with your feet apart or together – it won't affect how the deltoid works, but you may find that you get a little more back extension into the exercise with your feet together.
- Starting with the dumbbell in front of you, rather than at your side, let the supraspinatus muscle do its job (this little muscle in the upper arm is like a starter motor for the deltoids; it gets the arm moving before the bigger deltoids take over).
- As you lift and the weights reach eye level, twist the dumbbell so that the front end is almost pointing at the ceiling. This stops you squashing the tendon of supraspinatus against the humerus bone.
- A good way of judging the quality of movement is that you will feel the body-weight shift from the ball of the foot to the heel as you raise to the top of the move.

tricks of the trade

This move always seem easier if you do it in front of a mirror – I know it sounds a really simple suggestion, but it really does make a difference to how well my clients perform it.

exercise 11 bent arm pullover

• **stability** • **strength** • **power** • **integration** • **bench**

a
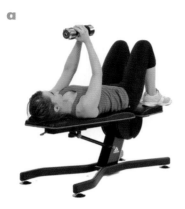

b
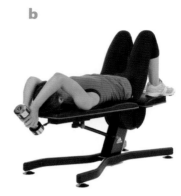

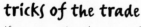

If you are doing this move on a step or low bench, then having your feet on the floor should be fine, but if you are on a full-size bench you might find as you take the dumbbell back that your feet lift off the ground, which is bad technique. Personally, I like to put my feet on the bench – that means I can't use my legs as a counterbalance for the moving dumbbell, and my legs will always weigh more than any dumbbell I'd be using on this move.

● Lie on your back with a dumbbell held in both hands and with arms slightly bent, above your sternum.
● Your arms and the weight travel through an arc starting from above the sternum and ending when the weight is behind the head.

tricks of the trade

If you practise the move first without the weight you will establish how good your range of motion is ('learn it, then work it!'). The dumbbell will just go out of sight as you lower it, which is the easy part, then you have to turn on the force and lift it back to the start position.

Remember this is predominantly a chest move so that's where you want to feel the force coming from when you pull the weight back to the start position.

exercise 12 straight arm pullover

• **stability** • **strength** • **power** • **integration** • **bench**

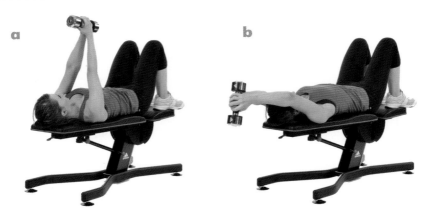

This move is more intense than the bent arm version (exercise 11) because of simple mechanics – as the straight arm is effectively a longer lever, the weight on the end of it will feel heavier. The same rules for the bench and where you place your feet apply. Again, practise the move first without the weight to establish how good your range of motion is ('learn it, then work it!').

- Lay on your back with a dumbbell held in both hands. Hold your arms straight above your sternum.
- The dumbbell will just go out of sight as you lower it, which is the easy part, then you have to turn on the force and lift it back to the start position.
- Remember: this is predominantly a chest move so that's where you want to feel the force coming from when you pull the weight back to the start position.

tricks of the trade

I see a lot of heavy lifters lifting their butt high off the bench. If you look closely this actually cancels out the movement in the shoulder and instead induces a simple pivot or roll on the back of the shoulders. They are still working muscles, but probably not those they intended. Put a towel between the knees and squeeze it throughout the move and you will be surprised how much your movement quality improves.

exercise 13 chest press

• strength • power • integration • bench

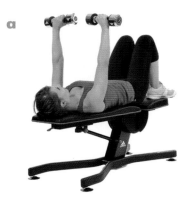

a

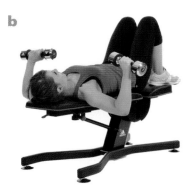

b

It is unlikely that you will chest press as much weight using dumbbells as you could with a barbell. However, if you set vanity aside, the dumbbell version will call upon a wider range of muscles because of the additional challenges placed on the torso to control these two lumps of metal as they move separately up and down.

● Start with the dumbbells above your sternum and the handles parallel to each other.
● As you lower the dumbbells, rotate them so that as they reach their lowest point they have gone through a 90-degree rotation. If you have a good range of motion then your knuckles should get as low as your ribs.
● When you reach the low point try not to 'push' with anything else like your buttocks; just reverse the contraction in the pecs and push the dumbbell back up.

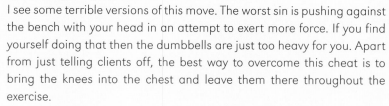

tricks of the trade

I see some terrible versions of this move. The worst sin is pushing against the bench with your head in an attempt to exert more force. If you find yourself doing that then the dumbbells are just too heavy for you. Apart from just telling clients off, the best way to overcome this cheat is to bring the knees into the chest and leave them there throughout the exercise.

exercise 14 incline chest press

• **strength** • **power** • **integration** • **bench**

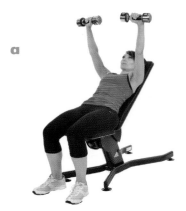
a

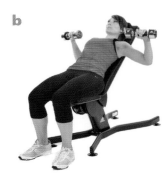
b

Most benches are adjustable between 30 and 70 degrees – any more or less than that and you may as well be flat or upright. You are using the incline because it will target the upper potion of the pectoralis major. Notice I don't say the 'upper pecs'; the pec muscle originates at the collar bone and goes to the base of the sternum, so it is one muscle that can fire different amounts of force throughout its span.

- Sit firmly against the bench and begin with arms bent, the dumbbells just off your chest, handles parallel to each other.
- Start to lift the dumbbells up. The starting position of this move is initiated by the triceps – which is fine, but if the primary targets are the pecs then you want to avoid straightening the arms until the highest point of the movement, so that they don't dominate the action.
- You will feel that the pecs are doing more of the work if you finish the move at the top with the dumbbells side by side rather than touching them end to end, which you achieve by rotating the humerus (bone in the upper arm).

tricks of the trade
Many personal trainers cue the client to keep their elbows in. There is no problem with this, but what actually happens is it inhibits the shoulder joint from going through its natural and strongest line of motion.

exercise 15 decline chest press

• **strength** • **power** • **integration** • **bench**

a
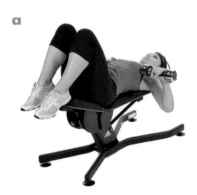

b
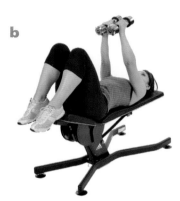

Since the pecs are such large muscles this exercise is really only going to be productive if the dumbbells are heavy, so you might find that an incline press-up feels more productive. However, this is a classic move so here goes.

- Start with the weights in the down position. Hold them so they are end to end. Your elbows need to be away from the side of your torso, or the triceps will just take over the force production.
- As you push up think about bringing your hands together only at the very top so that the pecs are active for the longest possible time.
- Finish at the top with the dumbbells side by side. Touching them together is purely optional – some people feel they are cheating if they don't, so you decide.

tricks of the trade

When I am training with clients I can help them get in and out of the correct position and hand them the dumbbells. If you are training alone, the easiest way of picking up and putting down the weight is to do it one at a time.

61

exercise 16 fly

• **strength** • **power** • **integration** • **bench**

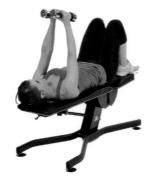

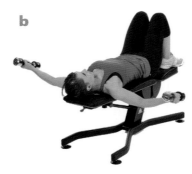

This move is more than a classic. It's not perfect because if you have long arms, the dumbbell is so far away from the fulcrum your natural instinct is to bend the arm more, which is considered bad technique. In reality, it's maybe just the wrong exercise for long limbed people.

Before you lift the weights know what 'good' looks like; go through the movement without any resistance so you can get a feel for your range of motion – normal is roughly when your hands disappear from your peripheral vision at the widest part of the fly.

- Start from the top, dumbbells side by side. Separate the weights so they arc out away from the body, your arms should be slightly bent throughout the entire fly.
- When you reach your full range follow the same arc back up again. If you get 'stuck' at the bottom, quickly bend the arms to bring the weights back in towards the centre line of your body.
- Remember, the pecs attach below the collarbone so this exercise doesn't involve the neck muscle. If you seem to be 'pushing' your head into the bench, then the weights are too heavy.

tricks of the trade

I find it helpful to give clients feedback as we train. For example, in this particular exercise the client should select the weight based on how tall they are and also how long their arms are (the longer the arms, the less light the weight). Keeping people informed makes the exercise experience more positive.

exercise 17 incline fly

• **strength** • **power** • **integration** • **bench**

a
b

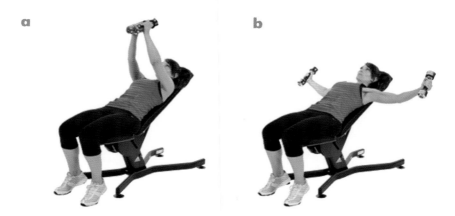

If the incline becomes too great (past 45 degrees), then this really becomes a shoulder press, so bear that in mind when setting up the bench.

● The same rules apply as for the incline chest press (exercise 14), but this time the triceps are completely left out of the move with the front of the deltoids taking over where they left off.
● You need to really keep control as you lower the weights. I see many people also rebounding off the bottom of the movement; that is fine, but I also suggest that you are going a little fast. The movement should look like you are drawing slow smooth arcs as you take the dumbbells down and out.

> **!**
>
> ## tricks of the trade
> Try this: when you brace your abdominals in preparation to push also push your heels into the floor – you will instantly feel more muscle activity in your torso.

exercise 18 decline fly

● strength ● power ● integration ● bench

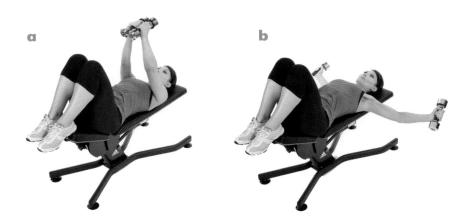

a   b

Again, this is really only going to be productive if you are using a challenging weight.

● If you think about how this move would look if you did it stood up rather than lying on a bench, then what you would see is a really big hugging action.
● The technique is the same as the fly on the flat bench (exercise 16), but the range of motion is less, so rather than the dumbbells going out of your peripheral vision they stay within it.

tricks of the trade

Think about the position of your wrists. Keep your forearm muscles engaged throughout the fly – this will help the biceps and pecs work together more effectively as a team.

exercise 19 seated bent over row

• stability • strength • power • integration • bench • ball

a
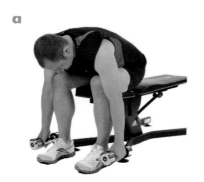

b
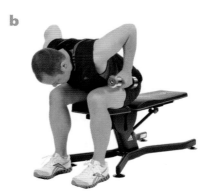

Clearly, being seated is going to switch off the work in the legs and torso that you get doing the standing move, so this becomes purely an upper body move rather than total body. This shouldn't necessarily be viewed as a negative as it just gives a different outcome. Use either a bench or a ball to sit on.

- Sit on the end of the bench with the dumbbells next to your feet. Check out your range of motion first by running through some repetitions without the weights in your hands. If your range is good, then the hands should come just a little higher than the knees.
- With the dumbbells in your hands, lift them up.
- It is really tempting to just drop them back to the floor, but don't: lower them slowly but don't put them completely back down on the ground.

tricks of the trade

Many clients seem to cut this exercise short by only going through approximately 80 per cent of their potential range of motion. To combat this it helps to raise the heels slightly: you can either rest them against the legs of the bench or place a block of wood or towels under them.

exercise 20 bent over two arm row

• stability • strength • integration

a
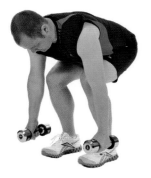

b
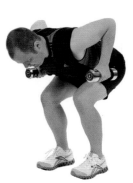

For this move to work the latissimus dorsi (widest and most powerful muscle of the back) you have to get into a pretty low squat position to begin. If you don't, this ends up being more about the arms than the huge targeted back muscles. Aim to look almost like a ski jumper in the tuck position, however, you don't want to get so low that your chest is resting on your thighs.

- Get into a squat position. Your hands should be in line with your toes and the dumbbells parallel with the feet. To fully lengthen the lats you need to have your shoulders rounded, but try not to hunch the shoulders up.
- Pull the dumbbells up towards the ribs so they parallel up to the legs.
- During the top end of the move squeeze the shoulder blades together (scapular retraction).

tricks of the trade

Some clients find the hardest part of this move is staying in the bent forward position. This position simply helps us to target the right muscle rather than being part of the challenge. Therefore if it is uncomfortable, stand up between every few repetitions – this is training, not torture.

exercise 21 hip hinge rear deltoid raise

• **stability** • **strength** • **power** • **integration**

a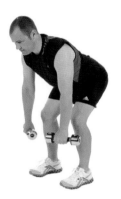

b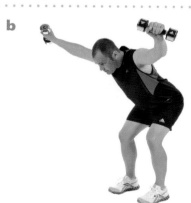

I didn't really start using the hip hinge stance until I began to understand the importance of core training. The hip hinge feels wrong when you first do it because unless you have practiced yoga or Pilates, then you have probably avoided this movement pattern. However, it is a good one to work on as it helps develop strength around the lumbopelvic region in a way that doesn't happen as soon as you push the hips backwards like in the regular bent over exercises.

- First, practise the hip hinge without any weights. If you have poor flexibility in the glutes (buttocks) and hamstrings it will feel like you are about to topple forward, so a good way to learn this start position is to do it with your bottom resting against a wall.
- To avoid targeting similar muscles as the bent over fly (exercise 19), your legs remain almost straight as you bend forward from the hips.
- When you reach the limit of forward flexion your arms will be hanging vertically. From there 'flap your wings', i.e. move your arms through a nice smooth arc, paying attention not to allow the dumbbells drop with gravity on the down phase.

 trick/ of the trade

Does your neck ache when you do this move? Yes? Try pushing your tongue against the roof of your mouth – this will activate muscles in the neck and stop the ache.

exercise 22 squat

• **stability** • **strength** • **power** • **integration**

a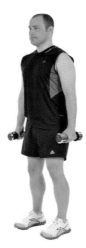

b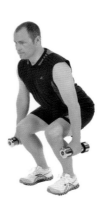

Clearly this is a leg exercise, but because in biomechanical terms the dumbbells are away from the fixed point (the feet), it means this move is one of the most total body actions you can practice.

Bear in mind that the load on the muscle is the dumbbells plus your bodyweight, so for some people that can really add up.

- Your feet really need to be no wider than your pelvis. Keep the dumbbells at your sides so that they run straight up and down rather than swinging.
- Bend the legs and squat down, holding the dumbbells on either side.
- I hear a lot of personal trainers constantly asking their clients to keep their heads up, but if you look at how the body really moves, it is more natural to look at the floor approximately 3m in front of yourself – why? Because the head weighs approximately 3kg and keeping it up actually means tipping it back, so it throws you off balance. Also, because you are going down, your brain really wants to know where it is going so it is desperate to look towards the floor.

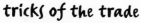

tricks of the trade

The big mistake many people make when they squat is that they bend forward rather than 'sitting down'. Therefore, keep the weight spread between the front and back of you feet and get all of the depth from bending the legs rather than taking a bow. With my clients I often make them stand close to a wall while they squat. By having their toes 30–40cm from the wall they simply cannot bow. It is virtually impossible to squat with the toes actually touching the wall – in 20 years I have only ever seen one person who could.

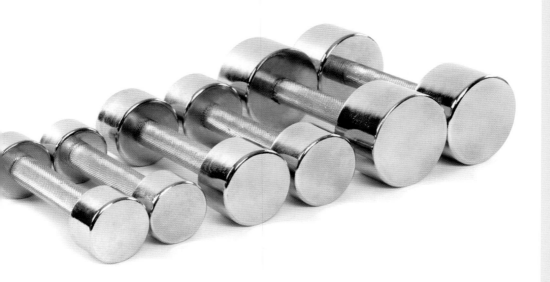

exercise 23 clean and press

● **stability** ● **strength** ● **power** ● **integration**

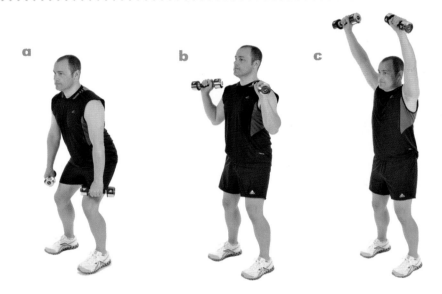

This move is more frequently performed with a barbell. I think this move is harder with dumbbells than it is with a barbell of the same weight, as while the bar is bigger, you will find having the weight separated in a pair of dumbbells requires greater coordination. Therefore, though performing a clean and press with a barbell can look more spectacular, treat that version as part of the learning curve to get good at the clean and press with dumbbells.

The barbell technique differs significantly to the dumbbell version, since you push your elbows and forearms under and in front of the bar, whereas with the dumbbells they stay down and to the sides. This is so you don't hit yourself in the face with the weights. Also, if you clean and press a barbell, you would start the move with the weight on the floor, but the bar stands much higher off the ground in the start position. Therefore, in the dumbbell version the start of the lift is when the bells are just below the knees.

● Sit down in a squat – the depth is achieved by sitting rather than bowing (see exercise 22).
● Hold the dumbbells end to end in front of your knees.

- Initiate the movement with a swift straightening of the legs while at the same time lifting the weights up to shoulder height (the weights travel the shortest possible route, straight up vertically). At this point, if you are using heavy weights you may need to pause and regain balance.
- To assist in pushing the weight up bend the legs again then, with a swift movement of the legs and the arms, push the dumbbells above your head.
- To get back down for the next rep, just retrace the line the dumbbells went through on the way up.

tricks of the trade

This move is the most effective way of safely lifting a heavy weight above your head but it requires you to commit assertively to the move – even when you are learning the move with lighter weights, make sure that you attack each section.

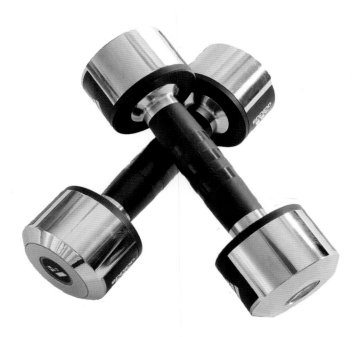

the best of the best

This entire collection of moves are certainly need-to-know moves, but you want to perfect the classics in the previous section before getting carried away with these more complex moves. It wasn't until the late 1990s that the fitness industry began to realise the importance of rotation (transverse plane of motion) for the development of optimal functionality and performance, so until then most of the classic dumbbell moves worked through the straight symmetrical planes of motion, known as 'sagittal' and 'frontal'.

This is another of those situations where the public could be forgiven for thinking that all personal trainers had suddenly torn up the rule book because there was an immediate tendency for trainers to squeeze a bit of rotation movement into all weight lifting moves, mainly for effect. However, I like to think that it wasn't that we were doing anything wrong, but that we were merely excited that we had just found the missing link for our strength programmes. Now the industry has embraced functional and core training you see almost the opposite situation: if an exercise isn't classed as being functional, then it will soon fall out of favour.

Some of the best of the best moves are also classics, so my apologies for mentioning them twice, but that's the thing about classics – you never get bored of them.

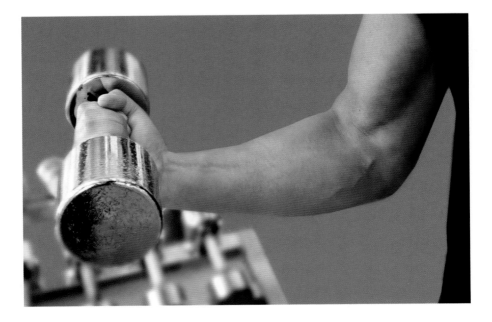

exercise 24 bent over one arm row

● stability ● strength ● integration

a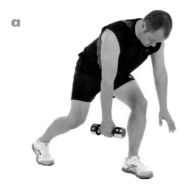

b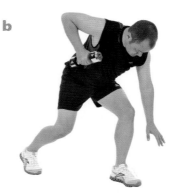

Doing this move with one arm allows you to really rotate through the spine at the top of the movement. This means that instead of limiting the muscles used, you maximise the recruitment of core stabilisers in the torso and pelvis.

● With a dumbbell in your right hand, stand in a split stance with your left foot forward.
● Lower the dumbbell towards the floor, keeping your arm straight.
● When you reach the bottom of the range of motion pull the weight up towards your shoulder, bending at the elbow, while at the same time turning your upper body (chest) away from the floor.
● When you reach the top of the movement the dumbbell should be in line with your chest.
● On the way back down don't just let the weight drop – I cue people by saying that on the way up they should try to feel as if they are rolling the dumbbell up their body and on the way back down they should unroll the movement.

tricks of the trade

Should the spare hand be on your knee? Yes and no: neither is wrong, rather just different. However, making the move 'hands off' will give greater activation of the core as it tries to stabilise the torso and pelvis.

exercise 25 bent over one arm raise

• stability • strength • power • integration

a
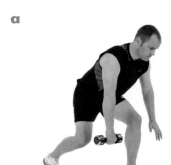

b
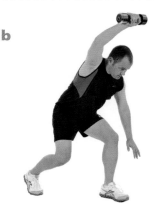

In my opinion, this is one of the superhero moves because when you do it, rather than being slow, controlled and compact, the bigger and more dramatic you make it the better it is. It may look similar to the bent over row, however, the feet are much wider apart because the dumbbell needs to come between the legs at the bottom of each repetition.

- Start again with dumbbell in your right hand and left foot forward in a split stance.
- The strength is coming from the deltoid, trapezius and a dozen other muscles. As you lift, a good mental cue to give yourself is that you want the raised working arm to finish shoulder width away from your ear rather than close to it.
- Lowering the dumbbell under control is hard as all your instincts tell you to just let it drop, but don't: you cannot defeat gravity, but try to stop it completely taking over.
- Let the dumbbell swing back into the start position and go again.

tricks of the trade

If there is one move that people suck the life out of it is this one. There is no need to keep the rest of the body perfectly still; it took us a long time to realise that rotation was good for us, so now we do, get some from the torso at the start and finish of this move.

exercise 26 bent over two arm raise

• stability • strength • power • integration

a
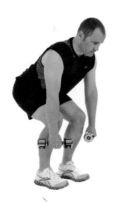

b
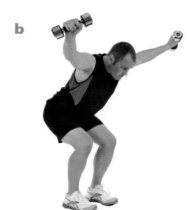

- Have your feet in a wide stance and turn them out so that you feel balanced.
- Lean forwards by hinging at the hips rather than rounding your spine and hang the dumbbells above your feet. Hold the weights so that they touch end to end, so you have made a right angle with them.
- Drive the weights through an arc so that when they reach the highest point your arms are in a 'V' above your head.
- The weight is now a long way from the support (your feet) so lowering them under control is challenging, but try to match the up and down speed.

tricks of the trade

This move will sort the men out from the boys (and the girls from the women!). When you first try this move you may find you instinctively want to stand up. There's nothing wrong with that, as instincts are good, but in order to direct the work into the targeted muscles you have to learn to stay down. A good way of doing this is to move the move before you load it so practise without weight, but also try it with your bottom leaning against a wall, as this will help you to condition yourself to stay down.

exercise 27 tricep dip, dumbbell in lap

• stability • strength • power • integration • bench

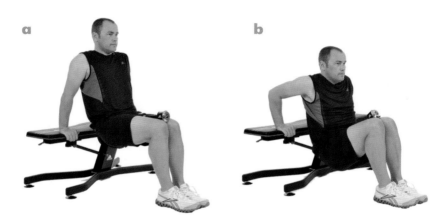

a   b

This move is a bit of a wild card, but if your aim is to target the triceps, then it is brilliant. It has the big bonus that it works the shoulder girdle in a very functional manner, which means that rather than isolating the arm to try and increase the intensity, we can also incorporate almost every muscle from the back of your head to the middle of the spine.

The height of the bench or step needs to be enough to accommodate your range of motion – you don't have to touch the floor with your bottom when you dip down. If you do go down excessively far, the nice 'pulling sensation' you feel on the front of your shoulder is the long head of your bicep tendon telling you that you have gone too far – so don't do it: listen to your body, it knows best.

- Sit on the edge of the bench, feet in front where you can see them. You now have two choices: keeping your hands close together will target predominately the triceps, or putting them wider apart will target the trapezius.
- Rest the dumbbell securely on your lap, push up with your arms then drop straight down until just before the end of your range of motion and push back up again.
- At the top of the move I really like to get a little extra squeeze from the muscles by 'depressing' my shoulders. You can only depress them a little but it works all those important muscles in the shoulders that you never hear about, like infraspinatus, teres major and teres minor.

tricks of the trade

Let's not waste our time here – I see people doing this move in classes and gyms with their feet close to the bench so that they can cheat and use their legs – get the feet out front where you can see them.

Obviously this move can be done without the dumbbell, but once you start doing it you will find the improvement is rapid, so adding the extra weight will have you doing less reps before you fatigue, thus quickly building greater strength.

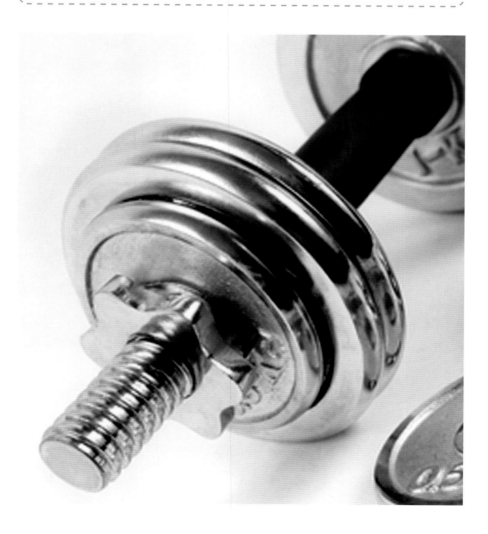

exercise 28 snatch

● **stability** ● **strength** ● **power** ● **integration**

a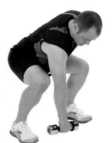

b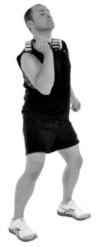

This is one of those moves where the dumbbell needs to be fairly heavy for you to feel where the 'work' takes place, but clearly techniques are easier to learn with lighter weights, so try to find a balance.

● Start with the dumbbell on the ground between your feet, your legs shoulder width apart.
● Squat down, grip the dumbbell, then quickly in one brisk movement get the weight to a position just above your chest to the side of your face.
● When you lower the weight back down, unfurl the movement in the other direction but slightly slower.
● Note: the force is predominantly coming from your legs, so don't hip hinge and just stand up (while this works to get the weight up, you won't be able to do it with a big weight so you'll be learning poor movement patterns).

tricks of the trade

If you have the mobility and flexibility to get into a good start position, you will be amazed at how much weight you can lift by attacking the lift. Also, this move engages hundreds of muscles each rep – if you are short of time, this one move is an entire workout in itself.

exercise 29 single arm hold/dip, dumbbell to reach

• stability • strength • power • integration • bench

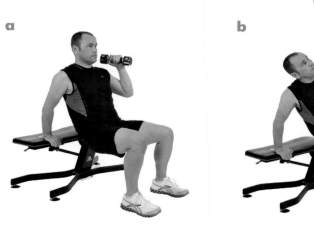
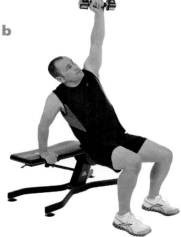

This move is more of a 'hold' from the triceps in the arm that is on the bench and a shoulder press in the arm holding the dumbbell.

- Sit on the edge of the bench with your right hand holding the dumbbell at shoulder height.
- With your left hand supporting, shift off the bench so that your body weight is loaded onto your left arm and both feet.
- Now, push the dumbbell straight up and at the same time shift your body weight towards the supporting hand.

tricks of the trade

This move works muscles right the way through the kinetic chain, from your hand down to the feet. However, people often say that this move 'finds' their weak spots, so it's often places like the inner thigh that stand out.

exercise 30 lying on side, front to rear raise

• stability • strength • integration

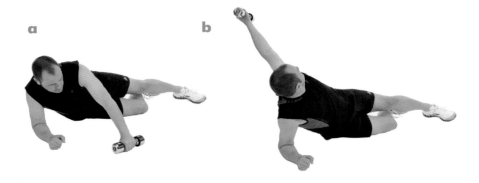

a   b

Be cautious when selecting your weight because it will feel considerably lighter in the front part of the move than it does when you reach behind.

- Lying on your side, split your feet with the top leg slightly in front.
- Place the dumbbell at arm's length in front of you and check that you have enough space behind you to swing back.
- Hold the dumbbell and let the top shoulder roll forward, then lift the weight up and move it through an arc above the body.
- When you pass the highest point decelerate the speed of the dumbbell and slowly proceed towards the floor (the best way I can describe the movement is that you 'open your chest' to get the full range of motion).
- You will feel that you are using your legs by pushing against the ground with your feet – this isn't cheating, rather you are simply engaging muscles throughout the entire potential network.

tricks of the trade

This is a move I rarely see in gyms, probably because I learnt it from working with track and field athletes. When you try it you will see why it is a favourite move for throwers, as it really asks the shoulder girdle to work in a unique way. Not sure if it is for you? Well, did you ever see a sprinter with poor shoulder muscles?

exercise 31 plank row

● stability ● strength ● power ● integration

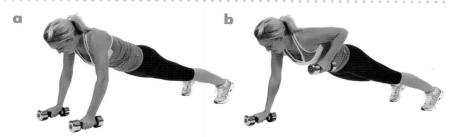

a   b

We have the world of Pilates to thank for this exercise because I don't seem to remember doing it before those guys started to appear all over the world. The plank became one of those 'must do' exercises and it probably took off because it was hard, rather than productive. I'm not a big fan of any exercise that requires you to stay still, which is why I like this dumbbell version because it adds two vital components that I like to see in my moves: lift and rotation. This move is a prime candidate for the 'learn it, then work it' approach, so practise the lift without the dumbbell first (saying that, I find that being 'up' on the dumbbells is kinder to the wrists).

● Start in a position similar to a press-up, but have your feet slightly wider, at about shoulder width. You need to have a straight line running from your shoulder via your hip through your knee and down to the ankle.
● From the start position first practise just transferring your weight from one hand to the other. You will instantly notice that you are also shifting the weight on your feet from side to side – this is good.
● Having mastered the shift add the arm row. Bend your arm and lift the dumbbell to head height.
● Because this is a move that involves the entire length of the body, for some people it can be more of a challenge of coordination than actually lifting the dumbbell, so adjust the weight to reflect this.

!

tricks of the trade

This move is so great I want everybody to experience it! If I have a client who can't support their body weight very well in the press-up position I get them to place their feet really wide apart – it doesn't look very pretty, but it works. This is because with the feet wide apart the vertical height between the hand and feet is reduced.

exercise 32 plank rotate

● **stability** ● **strength** ● **power** ● **integration**

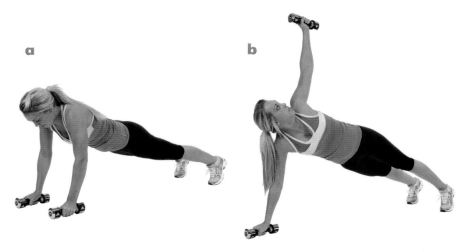

a b

A word of caution: this move feels so good when you master it that it is easy to get carried away, so remember that control is important.

- Start in the plank position (exercise 31).
- The objective is to go from a raised plank position to lift the dumbbell up. However, you want the dumbbell to travel the furthest route possible rather than merely being lifted straight up. So, think of a clock face. Your dumbbell is starting from 6 o'clock when you lift it; you want to take it through an arc right up to 12 o'clock, then back down the same way it went up.
- Don't go past 12 o'clock as the dumbbell suddenly feels heavier due to the mechanics of this move.

tricks of the trade
Movement is good, and the objective here is to get movement through the kinetic chain so don't feel you need to keep your feet still. As you lift the weight, one foot will have less pressure on it and because the hip is also moving, that leg will also move.

exercise 33 t-stand

• **stability** • **strength** • **power** • **integration**

a   b

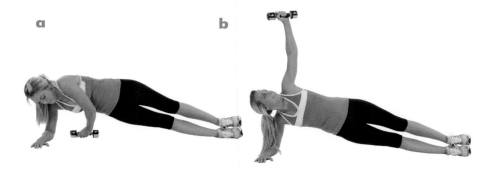

This is a logical progression of the plank exercises. The 'T-stand' in this move requires a similar approach because you are supporting your body weight between two points of contact with the floor, these being your elbow and foot.

Learn the movement using just your body weight as resistance before adding the dumbbell. Only try this move with a light weight, as when you reach the highest point of the movement the weight seems to increase because of the effects of leverage.

- Lie on your side resting your body up on your elbow. 'Stack' your feet on top of each other then lift the hip from the ground and find your balance.
- When steady, reach your top arm under your body by rotating through your torso, then unroll and reach up into the air.
- If you find this foot position uncomfortable then alternatively you can bend the knees (not the ankles). However, you need to bear in mind that this makes this exercise much easier because you have shifted the centre of gravity.

tricks of the trade

Hips tend to sag during this move. To overcome this, rather than think about using the waist muscles to keep you up, clench the much bigger gluteus maximus to bring the body back into alignment.

exercise 34 kayak

● **stability** ● **strength** ● **power** ● **integration**

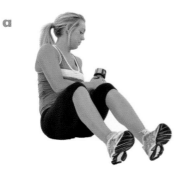
a

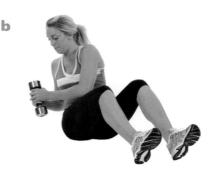
b

The name of this move is slightly misleading because when you paddle a kayak, the shoulders are doing far more of the work than during this exercise; visually, however, they do look like similar actions.

● Sit with your legs in front of you, knees bent and, most importantly, your heels pressed firmly into the floor.
● Start with the dumbbell next to your right hip then lift it up and over the body to the other hip. Arms slightly bent.
● Note: it is rather too easy to cancel out the exertion phase of this move if you don't really make yourself rotate through your torso.

tricks of the trade

A good indicator of whether you are performing this move correctly is if you feel your body weight transfer on to one glute at a time, rather than being evenly spread between the two. If you don't feel that much is happening when you try this move, separate your feet to shoulder width, then instead of placing the dumbbell close to your hip, reach a little wider.

exercise 35 toe touch

● stability ● strength ● integration

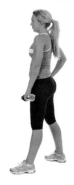

a

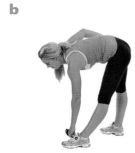

b

This move is as functional as they come. While we always have a little voice in our head saying, 'Bend your knees, keep your back straight' when we exercise, in reality the way we move is much more random.

● Stand with feet shoulder width apart.
● Holding the dumbbell in your right hand, bend down from the waist so that the dumbbell tracks parallel to the front of your right leg. Flexibility in your hamstrings will determine how low you can go, but all the way to the floor is your objective.
● You will notice when you are bending down that the right shoulder is lower than the left; this is because you are rotating through your spine. As you stand back up the weight will shift from the right foot back on to both feet equally.
● The up phase of this move is the most productive so don't creep downwards and then just stand up with no thought for the quality of your movement.
● Note: unless you are very flexible in the hamstrings, don't perform this move quickly because the benefits will be outweighed by the ballistic stretch that inevitably occurs in the hamstrings.

tricks of the trade

The 'best of the best' moves all have one thing in common: they all achieve multiple benefits. At one time, many of these compound moves proved their worth to bodybuilders and strongmen, but were then frowned upon by the mainstream fitness industry who shunned anything that didn't follow a single plane of motion. Thank goodness things have changed.

exercise 36 windmill

● **stability** ● **strength** ● **integration**

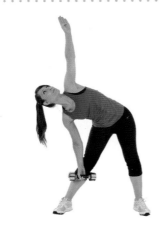

a

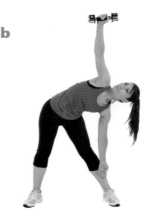

b

Today, strength training with kettlebells has a loyal following and I expect some kettlebell lifters would claim ownership of the windmill exercise. However, the main reason for using kettlebells is to move them at speed to work against the inertia, as we aren't building up momentum this move can be equally performed well with a dumbbell – weight is weight, it is irrelevant to whether the weight has one lump of metal or two. In reality though, I believe if you're moving, you're improving.

● The action is similar to the toe touch (exercise 35), but you are also going to lift the dumbbell above the head after the toe touch.
● As you reach down, the other arm reaches above you, the outcome being that you are transferring force throughout the lumbopelvic region.
● The up phase of the windmill is faster than the down because you are going to snatch the dumbbell up to shoulder height.
● See the photos: the most important part of the technique to note is the amount of side lean you need to recruit when the dumbbell is above you.

tricks of the trade
Most of my clients do better at this move if we go through 6–8 repetitions each side without the weight before adding the challenge of movement plus resistance.

exercise 37 cross chop

• **stability** • **strength** • **power** • **integration**

a
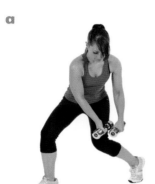

b
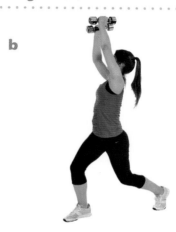

I see this exercise performed with driving force on both the up and the down phase, but I really think it is only safe to use force on the up phase because, with gravity lending a hand, you risk hitting yourself with the dumbbell. 'Learn it, then work it' because you need to perfect balance before attempting to move while swinging a dumbbell.

- Stand in a lunge position, your left foot back, but distribute your weight evenly between your front and back foot.
- You must rotate through the spine – turning your shoulder just isn't enough, so rotate around as far as you can with the aim being to lean towards the outside of the back leg.
- Once you have rotated to your full range of movement, bend both legs before you recoil and lift the dumbbell through an arc until it is in front of you and just above head height.

tricks of the trade

This move is so beneficial because the body is fighting against the acceleration and deceleration that occurs at the extreme ends of the range of movement. If you do practise this without a dumbbell first, then when you add the weight you will really notice the increase in velocity that occurs when you get that lump of metal moving.

exercise 38 ground to high chop

● **stability** ● **strength** ● **power** ● **integration**

a

b

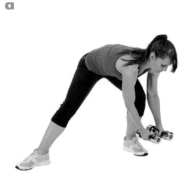
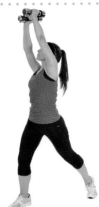

This is a great exercise, but it depends upon a good level of mobility to really get the full effect. One of the main mistakes I see with moves like this is that people seem to punctuate the movement, i.e. they bend – stop, they lift – stop, etc. What they should do is blend all the components of the movement together to make it look smooth. The other common mistake is to make the move too 'neat', so my advice is to make it look 'dramatic'.

● Start with the dumbbell next to your left foot, feet parallel and shift your weight onto your left leg (you will really feel this in the inner thigh adductor muscles).
● To get the dumbbell moving you need to push through your left leg and simultaneously lift the weight. The aim is to move it in a big semi-circle to the opposite side. As you pass through the centre line (12 o'clock), shift your body weight onto the right foot.
● As soon as you pass the 12 o'clock line you need to decelerate the dumbbell down to the floor. Gently touch the floor on the right and repeat, going back the other way.

tricks of the trade

The first time I teach this move to clients I get them to imagine the dumbbell is a paint brush and I want them to paint a really big semi-circle on the wall starting at one foot then finishing at the other – if you also think this way you won't end up taking the dumbbell through the shortest route.

exercise 39 squat, dumbbell at waist

● stability ● strength ● power ● integration

 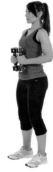 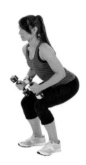

If you watch people closely (I'm a real people watcher) you can learn much about movement patterns. If they are carrying heavy items, they will keep the weight either at arm's length hanging down, or they will bring it into the stomach, or hoist it up to chest height and rest it on the top of their ribs. All these positions are very efficient and natural as throughout evolution we have adapted movements so that they become very effective at recruiting as many muscles to minimise fatigue on individual muscle and effectively 'spread the load'. Doing this move with a pair of dumbbells rather than a single heavy weight will give a slightly different sensation, however, the outcomes are really similar.

● Start by standing upright.
● Bend your elbows and hold the weight close to the centre line of your body so it's in front of you rather than at the side, which differs to the way you would hold it in the regular squat.
● Separate the feet to pelvis width then bend your knees and squat down, keeping the dumbbell tight to your body.

tricks of the trade

This move isn't really about 'lifting' the weight, rather it is about dealing with the effects of holding the weight – the knock-on effects of holding the weights are far greater throughout the kinetic chain than simply the extra effort required from the leg muscles to function with a few extra kilos onboard. Because you have your feet separated, you can get a good range of motion on the down phase. A good depth gauge is that your forearms should touch your thigh just above the knee.

exercise 40 squat, dumbbell at shoulder

● **stability** ● **strength** ● **power** ● **integration**

a
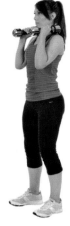

b
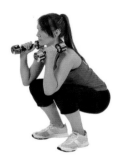

While this move doesn't resemble any everyday movement pattern, it is a very concise way of challenging and thus improving the strength throughout the kinetic chain.

As this is a leg exercise the weight needs to be heavy enough to be productive, however, you also need to be able to get those weights up to, and hold them at, shoulder height.

● Lift the dumbbells to shoulder height and stand with feet chest width apart. Aim to keep the dumbbells close to your shoulders and have the elbows out in front.
● Squat down until your thighs are horizontal then push back up.

tricks of the trade

When you squat down, the depth you reach is very dependent upon the flexibility in your calf muscles. For many years we 'accommodated' this problem by resting the heels on a support (normally a block of wood). However, now we focus on the functionality of exercise, I don't think we can still offer this option, as it is just a short-term fix. Substitute this for a few minutes of stretching the calf muscles every day and most people will see a huge improvement in just one month.

exercise 41 squat, dumbbell above head (prisoner squat)

• stability • strength • power • integration

a
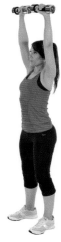

b
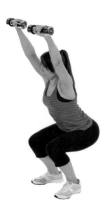

The purists out there might not call this a true prisoner squat because in that move, you have your hands behind your head, hence the name, as it looks like you have your hands cuffed. This move also bears a similarity to a 'Y' squat but, actually, it isn't that either because for this move I want your arms to be much closer to vertical than in the 'Y' squat.

- Set your feet into a comfortable squat stance then clean and press the weights above your head.
- Take a moment to ensure you are balanced and then squat down as far as you can without losing control of the weights.
- I like to alternate between having the dumbbells end to end and side by side, as this makes a very subtle difference to the muscle recruitment in the shoulders.

tricks of the trade

The eye line is the same as with other squats, i.e. look at the floor about 3m in front of you. Some personal trainers often cue their clients to 'keep the chin up', but this really throws out the balance for no good reason.

91

exercise 42 deep squat

• **stability** • **strength** • **power** • **integration**

a 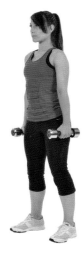 b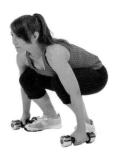

You have to approach this move with caution, not because it is dangerous, but rather I find that so few people ever do it you are probably new to it.

- Stand with your feet at pelvis width apart and hold the dumbbells at the sides of your body.
- As you squat down try to go as low as you can, it is fine to let the weights come a little further forwards than in a regular squat, so that when the weights get to the floor, they will be more to the front of the foot than the side.
- Some personal trainers habitually cue this move by saying: 'Keep the shoulders back' but logically this is wrong. Keeping the shoulders back is going to restrict how low you can go because to squat right down you must let the mid-thoracic region of the spine go into flexion.

tricks of the trade

When I train new groups of people, this move is the one guaranteed to send a gasp around the room. People have hung onto the notion that we should only squat down to 90 degrees, and when you ask them why, they say it is because any lower than that 'is dangerous'. Really? Squatting all the way down is totally natural and if you watch many populations working and resting they spend huge amounts of time in a full squat position. It wouldn't be advisable to suddenly drop down all the way with a great deal more than just your body weight without ever having done a deep squat, so those extra 15–20 degrees of squat need to be loaded progressively. If this sounds negative, it isn't meant to: I just really believe in the 'learn it, then work it' approach.

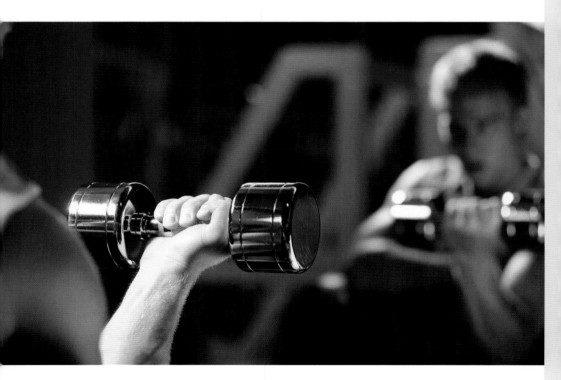

exercise 43 wide stance squat

• stability • strength • power • integration

a 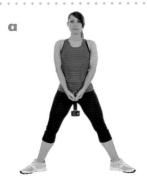   b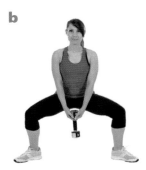

This is a great exercise for getting deep into the often neglected muscles of the inner thigh. While squats clearly do great things for the quadriceps, they also target the glutes and hamstrings, and in this wide position the adductors engage big time.

This move is best done with a single heavy dumbbell rather than a pair of mediums.

- Set your feet at elbow width first; stand with your arms stretched out to the side (crucifix style) then set your feet beneath where your elbows are, which will give you the correct position.
- Hold the dumbbell in front of you by the end weight rather than the handle, with the dumbbell hanging down vertically beneath.
- This squat is the only exception to my squat eye line rule, so this time you actually do need to keep your head up and look forward.
- Bend your knees to squat down either until you feel the other end of the dumbbell touch the floor or until your thigh bone is horizontal.
- You will have felt the adductors firing as you lowered, which is good. Now fire them again to stand up with also just the slightest hip thrust to bring in some extra glute activity.

tricks of the trade

I would suggest this move originates from ballet training. Dancers use moves like this to progressively develop phenomenal levels of explosive strength. With many of my clients, for every set of these I do with the dumbbells, I make them do another set without additional load.

exercise 44 wide stance squat, reach behind

● **stability** ● **strength** ● **power** ● **integration**

a
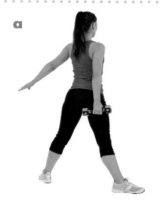

b
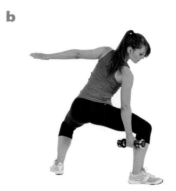

'Learn it, then work it', so do this move without the weight first to perfect the technique. You can actually perform this move with a pair of dumbbells, but I find that for most people one weight in the front hand is more than a big enough challenge.

● Set your feet in the wide stance position (the guide position is to hold your arms out to the side, then place your feet below where the elbows are).
● Hold the single dumbbell by the handle with the hand that is going to reach behind.
● Hold the weight behind you then bend the knees to start the squat; when you first do this exercise, you will find that you can get the dumbbell about as low as the back of your knees, but with practice it is possible to get the weight all the way to the floor.
● Push back up. Do all your reps on one side rather than switching hands for each rep (that would be seriously showing off and is not what dumbbells are designed for).

> **! tricks of the trade**
> This move is not supposed to look as if you are doing limbo dancing – to stop yourself from leaning back excessively, place the unweighted hand lightly on the back of a sturdy object to help keep you focused.

95

exercise 45 step-ups

• stability • strength • power • integration • bench

a
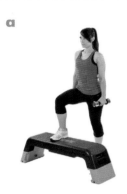

b
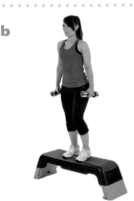

When I ask you to use a bench for the step-ups, I don't mean a weight training bench, since they are not designed to be stood upon (the combination of soft upholstery and their narrow profile makes them very unsuitable for this). If you are doing this exercise in a gym, you may be lucky enough to have a plyo (plyometric) bench (it looks like a low table). If this is not available, use a studio step or old-fashioned school gym bench.

Remember that when you do these step-ups you are lifting your body weight plus the weight of the dumbbells, so be sensible with your weight selection.

● Stand no more than a shoe length from the bench.
● With the weights hanging at your side, step up onto the platform with one foot, making sure that the whole of the foot is supported by the bench (don't allow your heels to hang off the back).
● Place the other foot next to it then step back down to the floor with the first foot.
● Do the full set of reps with the same lead leg before changing to start with the other foot.

tricks of the trade
The benefits of step-ups are seen when the bench is between 6in and 12in high. Benches higher than this will be most suitable for people over 6ft tall. This applies to stepping not jumping – benches for jumping can be as high as you can safely cope with.

exercise 46 single leg no pressure step-ups

• **stability** • **strength** • **power** • **integration** • **bench**

a
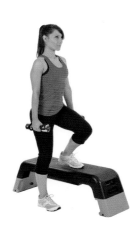

b
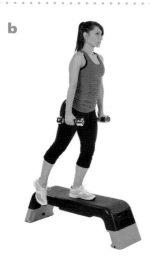

This is a completely different exercise from the step-up in exercise 45, in which you 'unload' the weight on every repetition. With this move the pressure stays on the working leg throughout the entire set.

- Place one foot on the platform (no heels hanging off please).
- Lean your upper body over that leg then push up, once you reach your full height rather than touching the trailing foot down, leave it off the platform.
- Then, without letting gravity completely take over, shift your weight as if to step back down, but leave the foot on the platform and repeat with the same lead leg.

tricks of the trade
Phew, this is a hard move and I often see it done badly. I tell my clients to imagine that they are in a vertical tube so they can't lean forward or back without touching the tube, which invariably keeps them nice and straight.

exercise 47 single leg squat from high

• **stability** • **strength** • **power** • **integration** • **bench**

a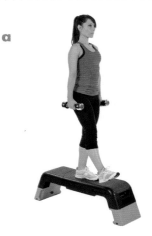

b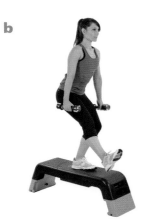

The biggest challenge here is not just giving in to gravity. I see some great attempts, and often people think they are doing it right, but actually they are doing a hip hinge rather than a squat, so keep that in mind.

- Stand on the bench with the working foot parallel to the side of the bench (you don't need to leave enough space for the other foot because you won't be placing it on the bench at any time).
- Hold the dumbbells so they hang at your side then bend the working leg. You will only be able to reach approximately 90 degrees before the biomechanics make it too tough to hold the position.
- As you push back up, remember that the single leg squat has been assessed as one of the best exercises to engage the gluteus maximus, so think of driving forwards with the hip slightly rather than depending totally on the quads.

tricks of the trade

I usually find that if you point the toes down on the spare (unloaded leg) then you'll get better balance. I think this is because the brain thinks you are searching for the floor.

exercise 48 single leg squat from low

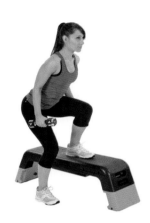
a

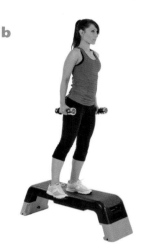
b

Everything about this move is the same as the single leg squat from high (exercise 47), except on the low version your hamstrings and glutes are going to initiate the move rather than your quads.

- Place the foot of the working leg on the bench and the other parallel to it on the floor.
- With the weights at your side push against the surface of the bench making sure that you stand up to full extension of the knee on the working leg.
- Don't just drop back to the floor: the combination of loaded concentric and eccentric muscle action needs to be maintained throughout the move.

tricks of the trade

Brace the abdominals before you start to push up, as this will help to stop the upper body being 'taken by surprise' as you push all that force through the working leg.

exercise 49 plyometric step-ups

● **stability** ● **strength** ● **power** ● **integration** ● **bench**

a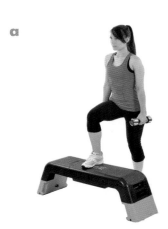

b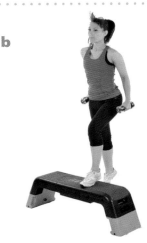

'Learn it, then work it.' If you can't do plyometric step-ups with just your body weight, then adding extra weight is just going to blow your chances of getting it right. You are looking to create a springy rhythm in this move, so rather than punctuating the different chunks of the action, your aim is to get them to blend together.

- Place one foot on the bench, lean forwards as you would if you were running up stairs, then push up.
- You need to be pushing hard enough to actually lose contact with the bench so you can change foot mid-air – so if you pushed up with the right, then you land with the left foot, hold the weights: however you fell will give you most control over them – either at your side or just in front of you.

tricks of the trade

You have a choice here when selecting your weights. For this to be a truly functional plyometric move, you want to be using the arms to gain extra upwards propulsion. If you go for a really heavy weight, this won't realistically happen, so this move is more about the springy action than the loading.

exercise 50 lunges stationary

● stability ● strength ● power ● integration

a
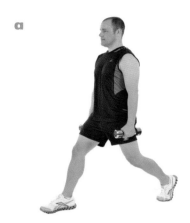

b
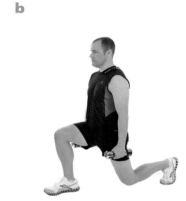

- For it to be a decent lunge your feet need to be well separate in a split stance. To do this it is best to shuffle both feet apart rather than taking one giant step with just one foot.
- Bend both legs so that the dumbbells go straight down towards the floor.
- You will predominately use the front leg on the down phase and the rear leg on the up phase – don't try and control this, as it will instinctively happen.
- When you have finished the set, shuffle the feet back together and change sides.

tricks of the trade

Under critique a lunge is a better functional muscle recruiter than a squat, but you don't see them performed anywhere near as often as squats (maybe you just hadn't realised how great they are!).

exercise 51 lunges front

• stability • strength • power • integration

a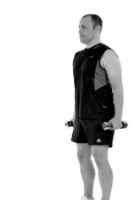

b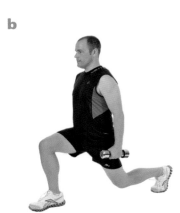

There are two phases of activity in the 'moving' lunges. As you step forward the supporting leg is doing the majority of the work; after you have planted the moving foot on the floor, that leg then becomes the force generator as you push back to the start position.

When you perform this move do not underestimate the amount of work that is going on above the waist – there is significant activity throughout muscle all the way up the chain to the ribcage.

As with so many of the best of the best moves it is best to practise this exercise without weights first, as you don't want to load poor movement patterns.

- Hold the weights either hanging down or lifted slightly to waist height.
- Stand with your feet side by side, your aim is to take an exaggerated step forwards. The length of this stride is dependent upon how tall you are, however, a good gauge is that you aim for it to be longer than a regular walking stride.
- When is a lunge not a lunge? When you don't go down. To perform a good lunge you must bend the legs to drop down, then push back up again. This might sound obvious, but I have seen many people just stepping forward and back without loading the working leg. The work occurs in two phases: there is the deceleration phase, when your foot makes contact with the ground, and the acceleration phase, when you push back to the start position.

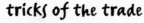

tricks of the trade

Movement in the upper body will alter the amount of load going through the legs, however, I don't think it should be completely discouraged. Some leaning forward at the front of the move will only encourage more muscle activity in the lower back, which frankly is a good thing.

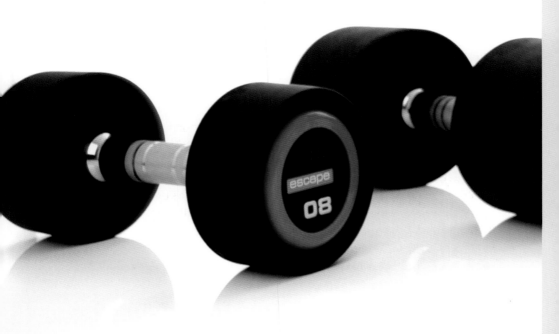

exercise 52 lunges rear

• stability • strength • power • integration

 a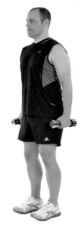

b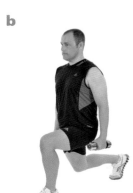

The same thinking applies to the rear version of the moving lunges, although you will feel that more work is being done by the leg with the fixed foot than you feel on the front lunge version.

- From your start position you are going to step back. It is possible to drop down and lose height during the unsupported phase, but it takes some practice to get that good – it's more likely that the drop down won't happen until you feel the moving foot make contact with the ground behind you.
- On the push back up press off the ball and toes of your rear foot.
- In actual fact, most of the work is being done by the supporting leg because you are holding the weights close to the torso.

tricks of the trade

There really is no need for the feet to stay close to the centre line as you step back – if it helps with your balance to separate the feet slightly, that's fine.

exercise 53 walking lunges

• stability • strength • power • integration

a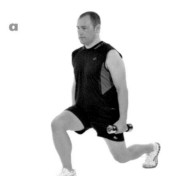

b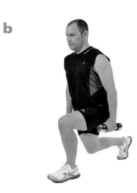

The only limitation of this move is that you need at least 10m of space to be able to get 5–6 sequential reps. The major differences between this and those lunges in which you repeat the move with the same leg for the entire set are that the force is being constantly transferred across the pelvic region, because you are walking and changing lead leg, and there is muscle activity happening from your fingertips to your toes, because the weights are in your hands. In short, this an awesome exercise.

● Practise first without the weights so that you get used to dropping your weight down without hitting your knee into the floor (never a good thing!) In your practice set you are getting a feeling for how long your stride can be: too short and shallow and it will look as if you are just walking, but too long and deep and you will probably get stuck at the bottom because you have over-extended your stride length.
● When you do this move well each step blends smoothly into the next, so try to avoid pauses. Make it flow and you will really feel the lower body working.

tricks of the trade

There is a reason this move is used in strongman competitions – it's hard. Strongmen perform this move (they call it the farmer's walk) with very heavy weights. Good posture is everything: as soon as you lean forward, it is very hard to recover, so keep your shoulders back!

exercise 54 plunges

● **stability** ● **strength** ● **power** ● **integration**

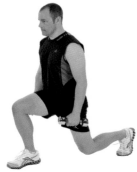

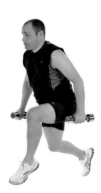

I don't know many people who would do this exercise for fun – these are really hard. My rule is that I won't do these with a client until they can do regular lunges perfectly.

A plunge offers a number of challenges to the body. First you have to accelerate as you jump up, then when you land you need to rapidly decelerate.

● Holding the dumbbells at your side, stand in a lunge position.
● You then need to introduce the intensity in phases; first practise switching legs quickly by dropping and jumping a small amount to swap the front and back foot. Then, once you are good at the fast feet phase add the depth.
● Unlike in a regular lunge the depth (or leg bend) occurs when you are in the air so you have already bent your legs before you make contact with the ground – hence the deceleration phase.

tricks of the trade
I really advise you to practise this without the weights first because as soon as you add speed to strength work, the exercises really amplify in intensity.

dull, but dependable

Not every minute of a workout has to be of earth shattering intensity and this little collection of dumbbell moves are *nice to know* – you won't be doing them very often, but for maintenance of some of the harder-to-get-at muscles they serve their purpose. These moves often come from the world of rehabilitation and are tried and tested. You can consider them to be suitable for injury prevention as well as useful for recovering from one.

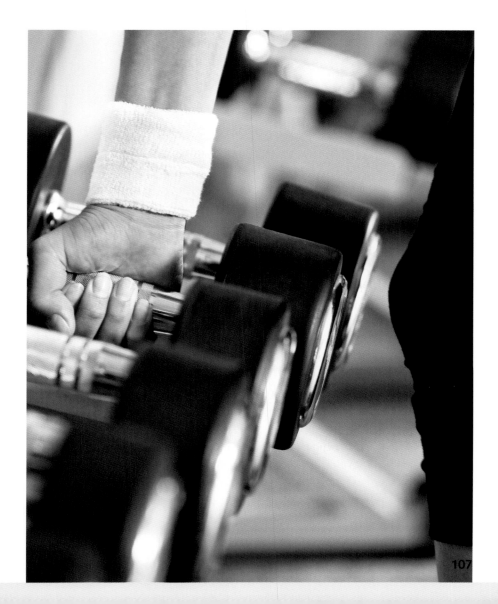

exercise 55 supraspinatus lift

• stability • strength • isolation

a

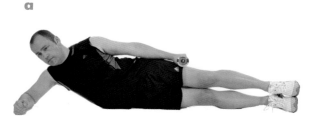

b

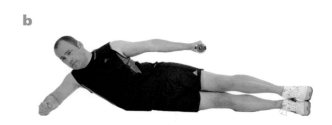

When aerobic classes became *the* fitness craze of the 1980s, a high number of the instructors developed a painful shoulder injury called 'supraspinatus tendonitis'. This was due to the fact that their teacher training taught them to 'keep the arms above the heart', which would 'increase the intensity of the workout'. I'm not going to get into whether that was right or wrong (it may produce the very slightest cardio response, but it is hardly noticeable), but bearing in mind that some teachers taught 20 hours a week, the constant arm pumping and shoulder pressing took its toll on the little tendon of the supraspinatus. Why? Essentially, supraspinatus is a little muscle that gets the arm moving before the bigger deltoid muscles take over – I often describe it as a starter motor. If you stand with your arms hanging beside you then 'flap' them just 15cm from your side, you may be astute enough to feel that it isn't the deltoids producing this movement, but the supraspinatus underneath the deltoids.

- To condition supraspinatus we need to put our body into an advantageous position. Lie on your side with the dumbbell resting on your top hip.
- With your arm parallel to your body, lift the dumbbell a tiny amount (approximately 10–15cm is enough).
- Then, keeping control, lower the dumbbell back down.
- Take a short rest of 3–4 seconds between each repetition as this muscle easily fatigues.

tricks of the trade

This is definitely an exercise where you'll get people asking what you're doing – just tell them that you are looking ater the unsung hero muscles of the shoulder!

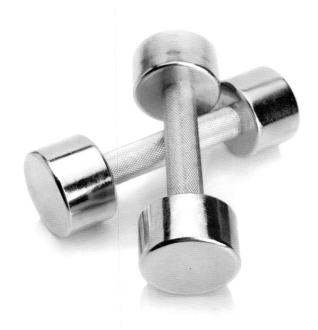

exercise 56 reach, roll and lift

● **stability** ● **strength** ● **power** ● **isolation**

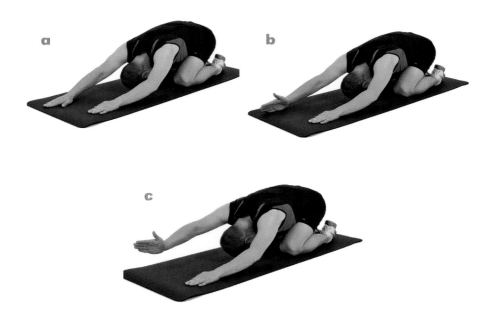

In a book that focuses on lifting weights this move stands out because it is the only one that you always do without the weight. This might sound odd, but the first time I do this with many clients they are amazed that they can even pick their hand off the floor, let alone a dumbbell. Many people find this movement challenging, so don't expect to be able to lift much higher than 10cm from the ground.

It deserves its place here because it manages to activate a range of muscles that don't get any care and attention during other exercises, but have to work constantly in every day life. These include the erector spinae, semispinalis and multifidi.

● Sit on the floor with your legs bent beneath you, shins flat. The perfect position is to have your buttocks touching the heels, but if you can't get this, don't worry: if you do this move often enough, the perfect position will eventually happen.
● Now lean forward as shown with your palms on the floor, chest on thighs and, if you have a good level of mobility, your forehead just above the ground.

- You are going to do exactly what it says in the title: working just one arm, **reach** forward by sliding your palm along the floor. When you have reached your limit, **roll** the hand through 90 degrees so that your thumb is pointing upward, then **lift** your hand off the ground.
- Lower that hand down and slide back to the start position.
- Repeat on the other side.

tricks of the trade

This exercise can almost bring big strong men to tears – it looks very easy, but I warn you now that it can take some practice to lift the hand very high. Don't give up: this move can really help you to have good posture.

exercise 57 circular swings

• stability • integration

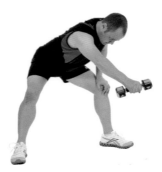

This is one of the few exercises that can genuinely be described as giving you a 'nice' feeling when you do it. This move has helped a number of clients over the years who have complained of non-specific pain in their shoulder, the type of pain that you can't put your thumb against and rub, or one that catches you during specific movements but just seems to be present all the time. These people are frequently new to strength training, so I think they have been simply loading their joints more than they are used to and, therefore, they've aggravated the joint.

- Select a medium weight; you're not really lifting the dumbbell much during this move, rather you are holding the weight and letting momentum create the movement.
- Stand with your feet in a wide stance and a single dumbbell between them.
- Bend your knees and rest the spare hand on your leg.
- Pick up the dumbbell and slowly start to roll it around in a circle. I cue my clients to imagine that they are slowly 'drawing' a circle with their thumb.

tricks of the trade

During this move there is a fine line between going too fast and grinding to a halt. If you get the speed just right it will feel like the dumbbell is being 'held' in place as it circles, rather than you trying to force it around the circle. I like to close my eyes while I do this – just because it feels so good.

exercise 58 standing calf raise around the clock face

• stability • strength • power • isolation

a 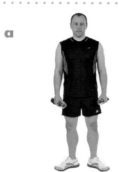   b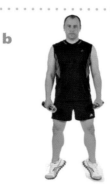

Many of the lower body moves are performed with the heels on the floor, which doesn't subject the muscles in the lower limbs and feet to specific periods of overload. A regular calf raise, where you stand with your feet apart then push up onto the balls of your feet, is a good exercise for the lower limbs, but I like to add an extra dimension to the activity by placing the feet in more 'random' positions. However, nothing I ever do is random, so in fact I actually walk the feet around an imaginary clock face on the floor.

The right and left feet are always opposite each other on the clock face meaning that if one foot is placed at 12 o'clock the other will be at 6, or if one is at 3 o'clock the other will be at 9, and so on. This process means that the calf will get worked more productively as the ankle will be flexed and extended while it is placed around the clock.

- Start with the feet split to the 12 and 6 o'clock position.
- With the dumbbells held at your waist, push up onto the balls of both feet.
- You might feel that you are more dominant on one side – invariably the foot that is slightly behind you will feel the stronger as it is working through a more favourable range of motion, however, because you are repeating the exercise on both sides, this will balance out.

tricks of the trade

There is no need to micromanage this exercise, so I find that using the foot positions 12, 3, 6, and 9 o'clock gives enough variety to work the calf muscle through its full range.

trash! don't waste your time

It's really easy to go with the flow and just do an exercise because you saw another guy doing it. But some exercises that are performed by countless people around the world are pretty much a waste of time or, if they're not totally useless, there is a different move that will achieve so much more.

I've been a member of more than 10 gyms over the years and as a personal trainer it is really hard to switch off and not be constantly thinking about the exercises that you see people doing right in front of you. Either you turn a blind eye or spoil your own workout by asking: 'Why are you doing that?' So by including this section I hope I can save you some valuable time because I have already asked the million dollar question about every exercise in the book: 'What does that move do and is there a different one that does it better?' While these moves are not totally pointless, you could probably spend your time more productively by avoiding them.

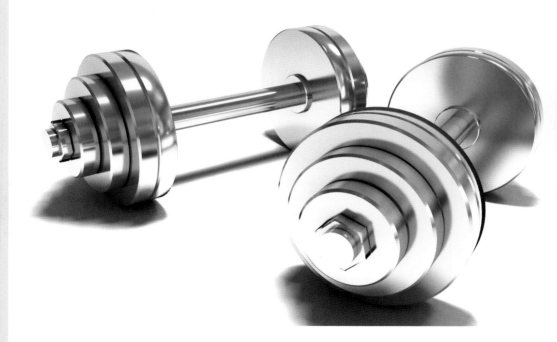

exercise 59 triceps kickback

a 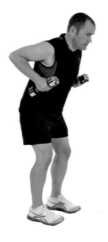   b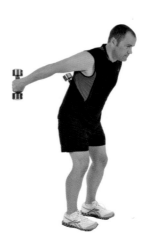

If you look at this move really critically you will notice that for most people the hardest part is holding the arm up in the start position. This is nothing to do with the triceps, but all to do with the fact our shoulders and arms don't extend much past 30 per cent, so the rapid fatigue stems from the position rather than the moving of the dumbbell (this is likely to be the reason I often see women straining to do it with very light dumbbells).

tricks of the trade

If you see anyone doing this move, do your good deed for the day and ask them why. Two much better options to work the same muscle far more effectively are triceps dips (exercise 27, page 76) or the standing triceps press (exercise 4, page 49).

exercise 60 side bends

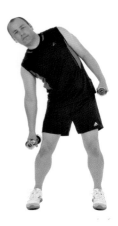

This is another favourite of the aerobic studio where dumbbells are often very light. If you look at this exercise you should notice that the main part of the movement is a pattern that we make all day long, meaning that the muscles are already conditioned to move approximately 40 per cent of your body weight through theses planes of motion. Therefore, adding a little dumbbell to the move will have very little impact. This exercise can be productive, but only when it is performed using a single dumbbell in the 10–25kg range held in one hand. To do this productively hold the heavy weight and lean sideways from the waist, the weight hangs on a straight arm and you would aim to keep bending until it reaches the height of your knee, you then stand up again.

 ## **tricks of the trade**

Despite this exercise being bad, there is a way of making it good. Stand on one foot, hold the dumbbell in one hand and bend to the side for 8–10 reps. Then, change hands (not leg) and do another 8–10 reps. Swap legs and start again. Alternatively, save your time and do the ground to high chop instead (exercise 38, page 88).

exercise 61 seated calf raise

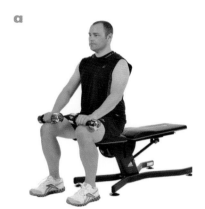

a

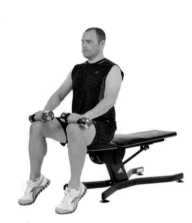

b

If your only goal is to increase the size of your calf muscles then this is a good exercise, but you will need to load the weights pretty heavy. The reason you fatigue quickly when performing this move is because the gastrocnemius muscle (the bulging part of the calf) originates at the base of the femur, so sitting with bent knees puts the muscle at a disadvantage. Also, this exercise really isolates the calf, which doesn't happen in real life because it is a 'team player' alongside the hamstrings and quads.

> ## tricks of the trade
> A better option would be doing the standard prisoner squat (exercise 41, page 91), then adding a calf raise the top of the movement.

exercise 62 weighted crunch

a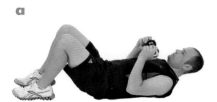

b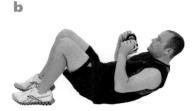

Crunches are fine, but there are plenty of moves that will give a more functional workout. The obvious place to hold a dumbbell during a weighted crunch is between the chin and the chest, however, that is right on top of the fulcrum of the crunch movement, so the weight is simply pressing down rather than being moved. A better place to hold it is above/behind the head, but that tends to make people sit up with a straight back rather than actually curl.

 tricks of the trade
Do the cross chop (exercise 37, page 87) instead – that way you will work the entire body, rather than lying on the floor and making your neck ache.

exercise 63 twists, dumbbell at waist

a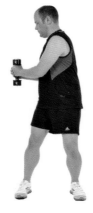

b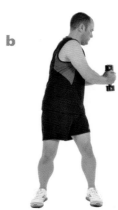

The weight is at the mercy of gravity, so only the biceps are working against a load. The rest of the movement is nothing more than an unloaded twist. The rotation may be beneficial to your mobility, but that's not a good enough reason to do this move as part of a workout.

tricks of the trade

Do the kayak (exercise 34, page 84) instead – it works because you have to lift the weight rather than just holding it.

3 training with dumbbells

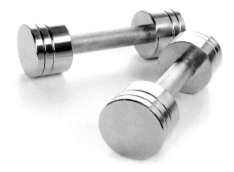

how to use the dumbbell training sessions

As people become more experienced in training with weights there is a temptation to forego a formal training plan and work through a session training body parts randomly. This can be effective, but human nature dictates that, given the opportunity, we often end up focusing on the parts we like to work rather than the parts we need to work.

The training sessions in this section follow the S.A.F.E. philosophy of progression and are divided into the three basic facets of this system: stability, strength and power. They are sequenced in such a way that if you were an absolute beginner when you started, you should have at least 18 months of progressive exercise experience before you perform the hardest session. So, a novice would first attempt the 15 minute stability session followed, when ready, by the 30 minute and then 45 minute sessions. This process could take three to six months. When the stability sessions have been mastered and no longer present a significant challenge, the 15 minute strength session can be attempted followed, when ready, by the 30 and 45 minute sessions; again, this process could take three to six months. Having developed stability and strength over this length of time the body will be well prepared to progress to the power sessions, which follow the same logical progressions. Note: the timings are approximate and include a short warm-up and stretching at the end of the session.

The reality is, of course, that many people are not complete beginners, so Table 2 gives you an idea of where to start depending upon your experience and physical ability.

| **Table 2** Assessing which training session to begin with ||
Stage	**Where to start**
You have not lifted weights on a regular basis	If so that makes you a novice – start with the stability sessions before progressing to strength then power
You have been lifting weights for 6–18 months and can do a perfect overhead squat	If so that makes you experienced – you might benefit from doing the stability sessions, but you can start with the strength sessions before progressing to the power sessions
You have been lifting weights for 18 months or more and can do a perfect overhead squat	If so, you might benefit from doing the stability and strength sessions, but you can start with the power sessions.

the warm-up

Before you start any of the workouts, you need to do a warm-up. This can vary depending upon where you are – in a gym you might choose to use the cardio equipment (treadmill, rower, cross trainer) to get ready. This is fine, however, I find the most effective warm-up is one that specifically mimics the work that is just about to be done, so I like to prepare by going through movements that feature in the actual workout, e.g. full range versions of light squats, rotation and shoulder movements, along with some temperature-raising activity such as jogging on the spot.

post-workout stretch

In the world of fitness we habitually stretch at the end of our workout sessions when the muscles are still warm. However, muscles will also be fatigued and therefore not particularly receptive to being stretched. The reality is that most people just want to get out of the door when they have finished the work section, and they view stretching as something that delays their shower, so I like to do the essential stretches just after the workout then make time when less fatigued to do some more quality, focused flexibility work.

The effects of stretching are cumulative so don't expect miracles the first time, or if you really struggle to make time for them, remember that the reason for warming up and stretching at the end of every session is to reduce the risk of injury. So, make a habit of incorporating stretching into your workout, or risk paying for the privilege of a physiotherapist telling you the same thing in the future.

You should complete the following essential stretches at the end of every dumbbell lifting session (see below). Hold each of the stretches for at least 20 seconds and try to relax and enjoy them.

stretch 1 down dog

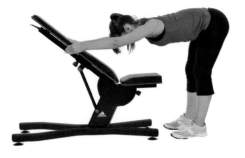

stretch 2 front and rear upper leg

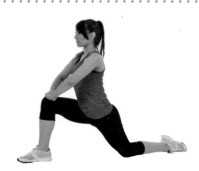

stretch 3 chest

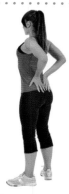

stretch 4 upper back

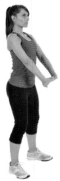

stretch 5 shoulders

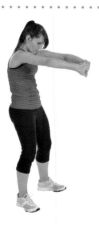

stability workout sessions

15 minute stability (15 reps per move ● 1 set ● 1 circuit)	
Order in which to do moves	**Technique**
exercise 39 squat, dumbbell at waist (page 89)	
exercise 10 deltoid raise side (page 56)	
exercise 50 lunges, stationary (page 101)	
exercise 19 seated bent over row (page 65)	
exercise 34 kayak (page 84)	
exercise 16 fly (page 62)	

exercise 8 dead lift (page 53)	
exercise 45 step-ups (page 96)	
exercise 4 overhead triceps press (page 49)	
exercise 22 squat (page 68)	

30 minute stability (20 reps per move ● 1 set ● 1 circuit)	
Order in which to do moves	**Technique**
exercise 19 seated bent over row (page 65)	
exercise 11 bent arm pullover (page 57)	

exercise 43 wide stance squat (page 94)	
exercise 31 plank row (can be done on knees; page 81)	
exercise 2 bicep reverse curl over grip (page 47)	
exercise 39 squat, dumbbell at waist (page 89)	
exercise 25 bent over one arm raise (page 74)	
exercise 45 step-ups (page 96)	
exercise 9 deltoid raise front (page 54)	

exercise 51 lunges front (page 102)	
exercise 17 incline fly (page 63)	
exercise 35 toe touch (page 85)	

45 minute stability (20 reps per move ● 1 set ● 2 circuits)	
Order in which to do moves	**Technique**
exercise 45 step-ups (page 96)	
exercise 13 chest press (page 59)	
exercise 34 kayak (page 84)	

exercise 20 bent over two arm row (page 66)	
exercise 52 lunges rear (page 104)	
exercise 4 overhead triceps press (page 49)	
exercise 16 fly (page 62)	
exercise 33 t-stand (page 83)	
exercise 22 squat (page 68)	
exercise 8 dead lift (page 53)	

exercise 9 deltoid raise front (page 54)	
exercise 51 lunges front (page 102)	
exercise 1 bicep curl, under grip (page 46)	
exercise 43 wide stance squat (page 94)	

Strength workout sessions

15 minute strength (10 reps per move ● 2 sets ● 2 circuits)	
Order in which to do moves	**Technique**
exercise 5 single-arm triceps press (page 50)	
exercise 23 clean and press (page 70)	

exercise 9 deltoid raise front (page 54)	
exercise 51 lunges front (page 102)	
exercise 8 dead lift (page 53)	
exercise 45 step-ups (page 96)	
exercise 12 straight arm pullover (page 58)	
exercise 22 squat (page 68)	
exercise 31 plank row (page 81)	

exercise 44 wide stance squat, reach behind (page 95)	

30 minute strength (10 reps per move ● 2 sets ● 1 circuit)	
Order in which to do moves	**Technique**
exercise 4 overhead triceps press (page 49)	
exercise 23 clean and press (page 70)	
exercise 10 deltoid raise side (page 56)	
exercise 47 single leg squat from high (page 98)	
exercise 8 dead lift (page 53)	

exercise 42 deep squat (page 92)	
exercise 13 chest press (page 59)	
exercise 37 cross chop (page 87)	
exercise 31 plank row (page 81)	
exercise 48 single leg squat from low (page 99)	
exercise 2 bicep reverse curl, over grip (page 47)	
exercise 34 kayak (page 84)	

exercise 33 t-stand (page 83)	
exercise 44 wide stance squat, reach behind (page 95)	
exercise 21 hip hinge rear deltoid raise (page 67)	

45 minute strength (10 reps per move • 3 sets • 1 circuit)

Order in which to do moves	Technique
exercise 23 clean and press (page 70)	
exercise 16 fly (page 62)	
exercise 27 tricep dip, dumbbell in lap (page 76)	

exercise 42 deep squat (page 92)	
exercise 30 lying on side, front to rear raise (page 80)	
exercise 14 incline chest press (page 60)	
exercise 2 bicep reverse curl, over grip (page 47)	
exercise 38 ground to high chop (page 88)	
exercise 12 straight arm pullover (page 58)	
exercise 26 bent over two arm raise (page 75)	

exercise 40 squat, dumbbell at shoulders (page 90)	
exercise 34 kayak (page 84)	
exercise 44 wide stance squat, reach behind (page 95)	
exercise 36 windmill (page 86)	
exercise 32 plank rotate (page 82)	

Power workout sessions

15 minute power (10 reps per move ● 2 sets ● 1 circuit min. 15 second recovery between moves)	
Order in which to do moves	**Technique**
exercise 8 dead lift (page 53)	
exercise 4 overhead triceps press (page 49)	
exercise 23 clean and press (page 70)	
exercise 20 bent over two arm row (page 66)	
exercise 46 single leg no pressure step-ups (page 97)	
exercise 28 snatch (page 78)	

exercise 21 hip hinge rear deltoid raise (page 67)	
exercise 49 plyometric step-ups (page 100)	

30 minutes power (8 reps per move ● 3 sets ● 1 circuit min. 15 second recovery between moves)

Order in which to do moves	Technique
exercise 23 clean and press (page 70)	
exercise 32 plank rotate (page 82)	
exercise 49 plyometric step-ups (page 100)	
exercise 28 snatch (page 78)	

exercise 13 chest press (page 59)	
exercise 34 kayak (page 84)	
exercise 38 ground to high chop (page 88)	
exercise 12 straight arm pullover (page 58)	
exercise 42 deep squat (page 92)	
exercise 29 single arm hold/ dip, dumbbell to reach (page 79)	

45 minutes power (8 reps per move ● 3 sets ● 1 circuit min. 15 second recovery between moves)	
Order in which to do moves	**Technique**
exercise 41 squat, dumbbell above head (prisoner squat; page 91)	
exercise 8 dead lift (page 53)	
exercise 49 plyometric step-ups (page 100)	
exercise 23 clean and press (page 70)	
exercise 13 chest press (page 59)	
exercise 54 plunges (page 106)	

exercise 32 plank rotate (page 82)	
exercise 28 snatch (page 78)	
exercise 38 ground to high chop (page 88)	
exercise 26 bent over two arm raise (page 75)	
exercise 12 straight arm pullover (page 58)	
exercise 33 t-stand (page 83)	

and finally...

Whether you are a personal trainer, sportsperson or fitness enthusiast, I hope you are now fully equipped to get the most out of the valuable time you spend working out with dumbbells. Dumbbells are an iconic piece of fitness equipment and they offer so many solutions to so many different training objectives. The possibilities are endless, and no matter what your goals, dumbbells can play a significant part in helping you achieve them.

All I ask is that you use all the information I have given in this book and make it part of an integrated health and fitness-driven lifestyle. My many thousands of hours spent in gymnasiums, health clubs, sport fields and with personal training clients has taught me that, given the chance, people like to do the things they are already good at. So before you reach your maximum potential training with dumbbells, the smart ones among you will be looking to introduce new challenges with different equipment like barbells, gym balls or medicine balls, as well as new challenges for cardiovascular fitness and flexibility.

The body is an amazing thing and responds to exercise by adapting and improving the way that it functions. Exercise is not all about pain, challenges and hard work, rather it is about making sure that in the long term your life includes the elements that have the greatest affect. Lift weights, walk and run. Eat healthily and drink water. Find time to relax. Stretch, but above all remember: if you ever find yourself lacking in motivation, the best advice I can give anybody wanting to feel more healthy is that if you're moving, you're improving.

fitness glossary

As a person interested in health and fitness there is no need to sound like you have swallowed a textbook for breakfast. Yes, you need to understand how things work, but I feel there is more skill in being able to explain complicated subjects in simple language rather than simply memorising a textbook. The following glossary sets out to explain the key words and phrases that, for a person interested in the body, are useful to know and will help you get the most out of this book, especially the training section.

Abdominals The name given to the group of muscles that make up the front of the torso, also known as 'the abs'.

Abduction The opposite of adduction (see below). The term the medical profession uses to describe any movement of a limb away from the midline of the body. So, if you raise your arm up to the side, that would be described as 'abduction of the shoulder'.

Acceleration The opposite of deceleration (see below). The speed at which a movement increases from start to finish. When using weights, accelerating the weight when moving it at a constant speed really adds to the challenge.

Adduction The opposite of abduction (see above). The term the medical profession uses to describe any movement of a limb across the midline of the body. So, if you cross your legs that would be 'adduction of the hip'.

Aerobic The opposite of anaerobic (see below). The word invented in 1968 by Dr Kenneth Cooper to describe the process in our body when we are working 'with oxygen'. While the term is now associated with the dance-based exercise to music (ETM), the original aerobic exercises that Cooper measured were cross country running, skiing, swimming, running, cycling and walking. Generally most people consider activity up to 80 per cent of maximum heart rate (MHR, see below) to be aerobic and beyond that to be anaerobic.

Age The effects of exercise change throughout life. With strength training in particular, age will influence the outcome. As you reach approximately the age of 40, maintaining and developing lean muscle mass becomes harder and, in fact, the body starts to lose lean mass as a natural part of the ageing process. This can be combated somewhat with close attention to diet and exercise. At the other end of the scale a sensible approach is required when introducing very young people to training with weights.

Personally I don't like to see children participating in very heavy weight training, as it should not be pursued by boys and girls who are still growing (in terms of bone structure, rather than muscle structure), as excessive loading on prepubescent bones may have an adverse effect. There is very little conclusive research available on this subject, as it would require children to be put through tests that require them to lift very heavy weights in order to assess how much is too much. Newborn babies have over 300 bones and as we grow some bones fuse together leaving an adult with an average of 206 mature bones by age 20.

Agility Your progressive ability to move at speed and change direction while doing so.

Anaerobic The opposite of aerobic (see above). High intensity bursts of cardiovascular activity generally above 80 per cent of MHR. The term literally means 'without oxygen' because when operating at this speed, the body flicks over to the fuel stored in muscles rather than mixing the fuel first with oxygen, which is what happens during aerobic activity.

Anaerobic threshold The point at which the body cannot clear lactic acid fast enough to avoid a build-up in the bloodstream. The delaying of this occurrence is a major characteristic of performance athletes; their frequent high-intensity training increases (delays) the point at which this waste product becomes overwhelming.

Assessment I like to say that if you don't assess, you guess, so before embarking on any exercise regime you should assess your health and fitness levels in a number of areas, which can include flexibility, range of motion, strength or any of the cardiac outputs that can be measured at home or in the laboratory.

Barbell A long bar (6–7ft) with disc weights loaded onto each end. Olympic bars are competition grade versions that rotate on bearings to enable very heavy weights to be lifted.

Biceps The muscle at the front of the arm. It makes up about one-third of the entire diameter of the upper arm with the triceps forming the other two-thirds.

Blood pressure When the heart contracts and squirts out blood the pressure on the walls of the blood vessels is the blood pressure. It is expressed as a fraction, for example 130/80. The 130 (systolic) is the high point of the pressure being exerted on the tubes and the 80 (diastolic) is the lower amount of pressure between the main pulses.

Body Pump® This is a group exercise programme available in health clubs that changed the way people think about lifting weights simply by using music for timing and motivation. Rather than counting the reps, the class follow the set tunes and work around all the different muscle groups as the music tracks change.

Cardiovascular system (CV) This is the superhighway around the body. Heart, lungs and blood vessels transport and deliver the essentials of life: oxygen, energy, nutrients. Having delivered all this good stuff it then removes the rubbish by transporting away the waste products from the complex structure of muscle tissue.

Centre line This is an imaginary line that runs down the centre of the body from the chin to a point through the ribs, pelvis, right down to the floor.

Circuit A list of exercises can be described as a circuit. If you see '2 circuits' stated on a programme, it means you are expected to work through that list of exercises twice.

Concentric contraction The opposite of eccentric contraction (see below). If this word isn't familiar to you just think 'contract', as in to get smaller/shorter. A concentric contraction is when a muscle shortens under tension. For example, when you lift a cup towards your mouth you produce a concentric contraction of the bicep (don't make the mistake of thinking that when you lower the cup it's a concentric contraction of the opposite muscle, i.e. the triceps, as it isn't ... it's an eccentric movement of the bicep).

Contact points The parts of the body that are touching either the bench, ball, wall or floor. The smaller the contact points, e.g. heels rather than entire foot, the greater the balance and stabilisation requirements of an exercise.

Core Ah, the core. Ask 10 trainers to describe the core and you will get 10 different answers. To me it is the obvious muscles of the abdominals, the lower back, etc., but it is also the smaller deep muscles and connective tissue that provide stability and strength to the individual. Muscles such as the glutes, hamstrings and, most importantly, the pelvic floor are often forgotten as playing a key role in the core. When I am doing a demonstration of core muscle activation, the way I sum up the core is that the majority of movements that require stability are in some way using all of the muscles that connect between the nipples and the knees.

Creatine An amino acid created naturally in your body. Every time you perform any intense exercise, e.g. weight training, your body uses creatine as a source of energy. The body has the ability to store more creatine than it produces, so taking it as a supplement would allow you to train for longer at high intensity. Consuming creatine is only productive when combined with high intensity training and, therefore, is not especially relevant until you start to train for power.

Cross training An excellent approach to fitness training where you use a variety of methods to improve your fitness rather than just one. Cross training is now used by athletes and sportspeople to reduce injury levels, as it ensures that you have a balanced amount of cardio, strength and flexibility in a schedule.

Deceleration The opposite of acceleration (see above). It is the decrease in velocity of an object. If you consider that injuries in sportspeople more often occur during the deceleration phase rather than the acceleration phase of their activity (for example, a sprinter pulling up at the end of the race rather than when they push out of the starting blocks), you will focus particularly on this phase of all the moves in this book. The power moves especially call for you to control the 'slowing down' part of the move, which requires as much skill as it does to generate the speed in the first place.

Delayed onset muscle soreness (DOMS) This is that unpleasant muscle soreness that you get after starting a new kind of activity or when you have worked harder than normal. It was once thought that the soreness was caused by lactic acid becoming 'trapped' in the muscle after a workout, but we now realise that this is simply not the case because lactic acid doesn't hang around – it is continuously moved and metabolised. The pain is far more likely to be caused by a mass of tiny little muscle tears. It's not a cure, but some light exercise will often ease the pain because this increases the flow of blood and nutrients to the damaged muscle tissue.

Deltoid A set of three muscles that sit on top of your shoulders.

Dumbbell A weight designed for lifting with one hand. It can be adjustable or of a fixed weight, and the range of weight available goes a rather pointless 1kg up to a massive 50kg plus.

Dynamometer A little gadget used to measure strength by squeezing a handheld device that then measures the force of your grip.

Dyna-Band® A strip of rubber used as an alternative to a dumbbell, often by physiotherapists for working muscles through specific ranges of motion where weights are either too intense or can't target the appropriate muscles. Dyna-Band® can be held flat against the skin to give subtle muscle stimulation, for example, by wrapping a strip around the shoulders (like an Egyptian mummy), you can then work through protraction and retraction movements of the shoulder girdle.

Eccentric contraction The opposite of concentric contraction (see above). The technical term for when a muscle is lengthening under tension. An easy example to remember is the lowering of a dumbbell during a bicep curl, which is described as an eccentric contraction of the bicep.

Eye line Where you are looking when performing movements. Some movement patterns are significantly altered by correct or incorrect eye line, for example, if the eye line is too high during squats, then the head is lifted and the spine will experience excessive extension.

Fascia Connective tissue that attaches muscles to muscles and enables individual muscle fibres to be bundled together. While not particularly scientific, a good way to visualise fascia is that it performs in a similar way to the skin of a sausage by keeping its contents where it should be.

Fitball (gym ball, stability ball, Swiss ball) The large balls extensively used for stability training by therapists and in gyms. They are available in sizes 55–75cm. If you are using them for weight training always remember to add your weight and the dumbbell weight together to make sure the total weight doesn't exceed the safety limit of the ball.

Flexibility The misconception is that we do flexibility to actually stretch the muscle fibres and make them longer, whereas, in fact, when we stretch effectively it is the individual muscle fibres that end up moving more freely against each other, creating a freer increased range of motion.

Foam rolling This is a therapy technique that has become mainstream. You use a round length of foam to massage your own muscles (generally you sit or lie on the roller to exert force via your body weight). Interestingly, while this has a positive effect on your muscle fibres, it is the fascia that is 'stretched' most. Foam rolling is actually rather painful when you begin, but as you improve, the pain decreases. Often used by athletes as part of their warm-up.

Free weights The collective name for dumbbells and barbells. There has been a huge influx of new products entering this category so in the free weights area of a good gym you will also find kettlebells and medicine balls. In bodybuilding gyms you will often find items not designed for exercise but which are challenging to lift and use, such as heavy chains, ropes and tractor tyres.

Functional training Really all training should be functional as it is the pursuit of methods and movements that benefit you in day to day life. Therefore, doing squats are functionally beneficial for your abdominals because they work them in conjunction with other muscles, but sit-ups are not because they don't work the abdominals in a way that relates to many everyday movements.

Gait Usually associated with running and used to describe the way that a runner hits the ground with the inside, centre or outside of their foot and, specifically, how the foot, ankle and knee joints move. However, this terms always relates to how you stand and walk. Mechanical issues that exist below the knee can have a knock-on effect on other joints and muscles throughout the body. Pronation is the name given to the natural inward roll of the ankle that occurs when the heel strikes the ground and the foot flattens out. Supination refers to the opposite outward roll that occurs during the push-off phase of the walking and running movement. A mild amount of pronation and supination is both healthy and necessary to propel the body forward.

Genes As in the hereditary blueprint that you inherited from your parents, rather than the blue denim variety. Genes can influence everything from your hair colour to your predisposition to developing diseases. Clearly there is nothing you can do to influence your genes, so accept that some athletes are born great because they have the odds stacked on their side while others have to train their way to glory.

Gluteus maximus A set of muscles on your bottom, also known as 'the glutes'.

. . . .

Hamstring A big set of muscles down the back of the thigh. It plays a key role in core stability and needs to be flexible if you are to develop a good squat technique.

Heart rate (HR) Also called 'the pulse'. It is the number of times each minute that your heart contracts. An athletes HR could be as low as 35 beats per minute (BPM) when resting but can also go up to 250bpm during activity.

Hypertrophy The growth of skeletal muscle. This is what a bodybuilder is constantly trying to do. The number of muscle fibres we have is fixed, so rather than 'growing' new muscles fibres hypertrophy is the process of increasing the size of the existing fibre. Building muscle is a slow and complex process that requires constant training and a detailed approach to nutrition.

Insertion All muscles are attached to bone or other muscles by tendons or fascia. The end of the muscle that moves during a contraction is the insertion, with the moving end being called the origin. Note that some muscles have more than one origin and insertion.

Integration (compound) The opposite of isolation (see below). Movement that requires more than one joint and muscle to be involved, e.g. a squat.

Isolation The opposite of integration (see above). A movement that requires only one joint and muscle to be involved, e.g. a bicep curl.

Interval training A type of training where you do blocks of high intensity exercise followed by a block of lower intensity (recovery) exercise. The blocks can be time based or marked by distance (in cardio training). Interval training is highly beneficial to both athletes and fitness enthusiasts as it allows them to subject their body to high intensity activity in short achievable bursts.

Intra-abdominal pressure (IAP) An internal force that assists in the stabilisation of the lumber spine. This relates to the collective effects of pressure exerted on the structures of the diaphragm, transversus abdominis, multifidi and the pelvic floor.

Kinesiology The scientific study of the movement of our anatomical structure. It was only in the 1960s with the creation of fixed weight machines that we started to isolate individual muscles and work them one at a time. This is a step backwards in terms of kinesiology because in real life a single muscle rarely works in isolation.

Kinetic chain The series of reactions/forces throughout the nerves, bones, muscles, ligaments and tendons when the body moves or has a force applied against it.

Kyphosis Excessive curvature of the human spine. This can range from being a little bit round shouldered to being in need of corrective surgery.

Lactic acid A by-product of muscle contractions. If lactic acid reaches a level higher than that which the body can quickly clear from the blood stream, the person has reached their anaerobic threshold. Training at high intensity has the effect of delaying the point at which lactic acid levels cause fatigue.

Latissimus dorsi Two triangular-shaped muscles that run from the top of the neck and spine to the back of the upper arm and all the way into the lower back, also known as 'the lats'.

Ligaments Connective tissues that attach bone to bone or cartilage to bone. They have fewer blood vessels passing through them than muscles, which makes them whiter (they look like gristle) and also slower to heal.

Lordosis Excessive curvature of the lower spine. Mild cases that are diagnosed early can often be resolved through core training and by working on flexibility with exercises best prescribed by a physiotherapist.

Massage Not just for pleasure or relaxation, this can speed up recovery and reduce discomfort after a hard training session. Massage can help maintain range of motion in joints and reduce mild swelling caused by injury related inflammation.

Magnesium An essential mineral that plays a role in over 300 processes in the body including in the cardiovascular system and tissue repair.

Maximum heart rate (MHR) The highest number of times the heart can contract (or beat) in one minute. A very approximate figure can be obtained for adults by using the following formula: 220 — current age = MHR. Athletes often exceed this guideline, but only because they have progressively pushed themselves and increased their strength over time.

Medicine ball Traditionally this was a leather ball packed with fibre to make it heavy. Modern versions are solid rubber or filled with a heavy gel.

Mobility The ability of a joint to move freely through a range of motion. Mobility is very important because if you have restricted joint mobility and with exercise you start to load that area with weights, the chances are that you will compound the problem.

Muscular endurance (MSE) The combination of strength and endurance. The ability to perform many repetitions against a given resistance for a prolonged period. In strength training any more than 12 reps is considered MSE.

Negative-resistance training (NRT) Resistance training in which the muscles lengthen while still under tension. Lowering a barbell, bending down and running downhill are all examples. It is felt that this type of training will increase muscle size more quickly than other types of training, but if you only ever do NRT you won't be training the body to develop usable functional strength.

Obliques The muscles on both sides of the abdomen that rotate and flex the torso. Working these will have no effect on 'love handles', which is fat that sits above, but is not connected to, the obliques.

Origin All muscles are attached to bone or others muscles by tendons or fascia. The end of the muscle which is not moved during a contraction is the origin, with the moving end being called the insertion. Note that some muscles have more than one origin and insertion.

Overtraining Excessive amounts of exercise, intensity, or both volume and intensity of training, resulting in fatigue, illness, injury and/or impaired performance. Overtraining can occur in individual parts of the body or throughout, which is a good reason for keeping records of the training you do so you can see if patterns of injuries relate to certain times or types of training you do throughout the year.

Patience With strength training – more than any other type of exercise – patience is essential. When you exercise the results are based on the ability of the body to 'change', which includes changes in the nervous system as well as progressive improvements in the soft tissues (muscles, ligaments and tendons). While it is not instantly obvious why patience is so important, it becomes clearer when you consider how, for example, the speed of change differs in the blood rich muscles at a faster rate than the more avascular ligaments and tendons. Improvements take time so be patient.

Pectorals The muscles of the chest, also known as 'the pecs'. Working the pecs will have a positive effect on the appearance of the chest, however, despite claims, it is unlikely that working the pecs will have any effect on the size of female breasts although it can make them feel firmer if the muscle tone beneath them is increased.

Pelvic floor (PF) Five layers of muscle and connective tissue at the base of the torso. The male and female anatomy differs in this area, however strength and endurance is essential in the PF for both men and women if you are to attain maximum strength in the core. Most of the core training or stability products work the PF.

Periodisation Sums up the difference between a long-term strategy and short-term gains. Periodisation is where you plan to train the body for different outcomes throughout a year or longer. The simplest version of this method would be where a track athlete worked on muscle strength and growth during the winter and then speed and maintenance of muscle endurance during the summer racing session.

Planes of motion The body moves through three planes of motion. Sagittal describes all the forward and back movement; frontal describes the side to side movements; and transverse describes the rotational movements. In everyday life most of the movements we go through involve actions from all three planes all of the time – it is really only 'artificial' techniques, such as bicep curls and deltoid raises, that call upon just one plane at a time.

Plyometrics An explosive movement practised by athletes, for example, two-footed jumps over hurdles. This is not for beginners or those with poor levels of flexibility and/or a limited range of motion.

Prone Lying face down, also the standard description of exercises performed from a lying face down position. The opposite of supine (see below).

Protein A vital nutrient that needs to be consumed every day. Carbohydrates provide your body with energy, while protein helps your muscles to recover and repair more quickly after exercise. Foods high in protein include whey protein,

. . . .

which is a by-product of the dairy industry and is consumed as a shake, fish, chicken, eggs, dairy produce (such as milk, cheese and yoghurt), beef and soya.

Increased activity will increase your protein requirements. A lack of quality protein can result in loss of muscle tissue and tone, a weaker immune system, slower recovery and lack of energy. The protein supplements industry has developed many convenient methods for consuming protein in the form of powders, shakes and food bars, most of which contain the most easily digested and absorbable type of protein, whey protein.

Pyramid A programming method for experienced weight trainers. A set of the same exercises are performed at least three times, each set has progressively fewer repetitions in it, but greater resistance. When you reach the peak of the pyramid (heaviest weight) you then perform the same three sets again in reverse order. For example, going up the pyramid would ask for 15 reps with 10kg, 10 reps with 15kg, 5 reps with 20kg. Going down the pyramid would require 10 reps with 15kg, 15 reps with 10kg.

Quadriceps The groups of muscles at the front of the thighs, also known as 'the quads'. They are usually the first four muscle names that personal trainers learn, but in case you have forgotten the four are: vastus intermedius, rectus femoris (that's the one that's also a hip flexor), vastus lateralis and vastus medialis.

Range of motion (ROM) The degree of movement that occurs at one of the body's joints. Without physio equipment it is difficult to measure a joint precisely, however, you can easily compare the shoulder, spine, hip, knee and ankle on the left side with the range of motion of the same joints on the right side.

Reebok Core Board® A stability product that you predominately stand on. The platform has a central axis which creates a similar experience to using a wobble board, however the Reebok Core Board® also rotates under tension so you can train against torsion and recoil.

Recoil The elastic characteristic of muscle when 'stretched' to return the body parts back to the start positions after a dynamic movement.

Recovery/rest The period when not exercising and the most important component of any exercise programme. It is only during rest periods that the body adapts to previous training loads and rebuilds itself to be stronger, thereby facilitating improvement. Rest is therefore vitally important for progression.

Repetitions How many of each movement you do, also known as 'reps'. On training programmes you will have see three numerical figures that you need to understand – reps, sets and circuits.

Repetition max (RM) The maximum load that a muscle or muscle group can lift. Establishing your 1RM can help you select the right amount of weight for different exercises and it is also a good way of monitoring progress.

Resistance training Any type of training with weights, including gym machines, barbells and dumbbells and bodyweight exercises.

Resting heart rate (RHR) The number of contractions (heartbeats) per minute when at rest. The average RHR for an adult is approx 72BPM, but for athletes it can be much lower.

Scapula retraction Not literally 'pulling your shoulders back', but that is a good cue to use to get this desired effect. Many people develop rounded shoulders, which when lifting weights puts them at a disadvantage because the scapular cannot move freely, so by lifting the ribs and squeezing the shoulder blades back the shoulder girdle is placed in a good lifting start position.

Sciatica Layman's term for back pain which radiates through the spine, buttocks and hamstrings. Usually due to pressure on the sciatic nerve being shortened, which runs from the lower back and down the legs, rather than being a problem with the skeleton. Most often present in people who sit a lot. Core training, massage and flexibility exercises can frequently cure the problem.

Set A block of exercises usually put together to work an area of the body to the point of fatigue, so if you were working legs you may do squats, lunges and calf raises straight after each other, then repeat them again for a second 'set'.

Speed, agility and quickness (SAQ)® Although in fact a brand name, this has become the term used to describe a style of exercises or drills which are designed to improve speed, agility and quickness. Very athletic and dynamic, often including plyometric movements.

Stability ball (also gym ball, fitball and Swiss ball) The large balls extensively used for suitability training by therapists and in gyms. They are available in sizes 55–75cm. If you are using them for weight training always remember to add your weight and the dumbbell weight together to make sure the total weight doesn't exceed the safety limit of the ball.

Stretch A balanced approach to stretching is one of the most important elements of feeling good and reducing the likelihood of developing non-trauma soft tissue injuries. When we lift weight clearly the muscle fatigues and as a result at the end of the session the overall muscle (rather than individual fibres) can feel 'tight' or shortened. Doing a stretch will help return the muscle to its pre-exercise state. Dynamic stretching (rhythmic movements to promote optimum range of movement from muscle/joints) should be performed pre-workout. Static stretching performed after the weights session is productive as long as you dedicate enough time to each position, so give each section of the body worked at least 90 seconds of attention.

Suspension training A strength training format that allows you to use your body weight as the resistance by means of hanging from long adjustable straps that are suspended above head height, also known as 'TRX®'. By adjusting the length of the straps and changing the body and foot position the challenge can be adapted for all levels of ability.

Superset Similar to a set, but each sequential exercise is performed with no rest in between. The moves in a superset are selected to ensure that they relate to each other, for example, an exercise that focused on shoulders and triceps, such as a shoulder press, would be followed by another shoulder/triceps move, such as dips.

Supine Lying face up, also the standard description of exercises performed from a lying face up position. The opposite of prone (see above).

Tendon Connective tissue that attaches muscles to bones. Muscle and tendon tissue merge together progressively, rather than there being a clear line where tendon starts and muscle finishes. Like ligaments, a tendon has a lesser number of blood vessels running through it and is less flexible than muscle tissue.

Time As a personal trainer, I have been asked many times, 'What is the best time of day to exercise?' The answer depends. If you are an athlete training almost every day perhaps twice a day, then I would say that strength training in the morning could be more productive than at other times due to the body clock and fluctuating hormone levels throughout the day. However, if the question is asked

be a casual exerciser with an average diet and a job and busy lifestyle, my answer would be to exercise at any time of the day, as exercise is a productive use of your valuable free time.

Torsion stress on the body when external forces twist it about the spinal axis.

Training partner A training partner can be a person who keeps you company and motivates you while you exercise or they can also take the role of being your 'spotter' when you are lifting heavy weights. The role of a spotter is to hand to and take the weights from you when you are fatigued from a heavy set of lifts. Choose your partner wisely; weights can be dangerous, so ensure they take the responsibility seriously.

Training shoes The best shoes to wear when lifting weights will have a combination of good grip and stability. Some athletes are now choosing to lift while wearing no or very thin soled shoes on the basis that it will work the muscles in their feet more and therefore give greater results – if you do consider doing this take a number of weeks to build up the amount you do barefoot to give the feet time to strengthen slowly. Athletes competing in powerlifting contests will wear performance shoes that give their feet increased support, however these are not suitable for exercises in which the foot is moved.

Transversus abdominis A relatively thin sheet of muscle which wraps around the torso. This is the muscle that many people think they activate by following the instruction of 'pull your stomach in', however that movement is more likely to be facilitated by the main abdominals. For your information, a flat stomach is more likely to be achieved by simply standing up straight, as this ensures the correct distance between the ribs and pelvis.

Triceps Muscles at the back of the upper arms. They make up approximately two-thirds of the diameter of the upper arm, so if arm size is your goal, working the triceps will be a priority.

Vertebrae Individual bones that make up the spinal column. The intervertebral discs that sit between them are there to keep the vertebrae separated, cushion the spine and protect the spinal cord.

VO$_2$ max The highest volume of oxygen a person can infuse into their blood during exercise. A variety of calculations or tests can be used to establish your

VO_2 max; these include measuring the heart rate during and post aerobic activity. As each of these tests includes a measurement of the distance covered as well as the heart's reaction to activity, the most popular methods of testing VO_2 max are running, stepping, swimming or cycling for a set time and distance.

Warm-up The first part of any workout session that is intended to prepare the body for the exercise ahead of it. I find it is best to take the lead from the sports world and base the warm-up exactly on the movements you will do in the session. So if you are about to do weights rather than jog, go through some of the movements unloaded to prepare the body for the ranges of motion you will later be doing loaded.

Warm-down The slowing down or controlled recovery period after a workout session. A warm-down can include low level cardio work to return the heart rate to a normal speed as well as stretching and relaxation.

Wobble board A circular wooden disc that you stand on with a hemisphere on one side. Originally used just by physiotherapists, they are now common in gyms and are used for stability training, core exercises and strengthening the ankle and/or rehabilitation from ankle injuries. Technology has been applied to this simple piece of equipment and you now have progressive devices such as the Reebok Core Board® and the BOSU® (Both sides up), which achieve the same and more than the wooden versions.

X-training, activity. See cross training (above).

Yoga Probably the oldest form of fitness training in existence. Yoga has many different types (or styles) ranging from very passive stretching techniques through to explosive and dynamic style. It is often associated with hippy culture and 'yummy mummies', however, if you are doing any type of strength training, yoga will compliment this nicely.

about the author

STEVE BARRETT is a former national competitor in athletics, rugby, mountain biking and sport aerobics. His career in the fitness industry as a personal trainer spans over 20 years. His work as a lecturer and presenter has taken him to 32 countries including the United States, Russia and Australia.

For many years Steve delivered Reebok International's fitness strategy and implementation via their training faculty Reebok University. He gained the title of Reebok Global Master Trainer, which is a certification that required a minimum of three years' studying, presenting and researching both practical and academic subjects. Between the years 2000 and 2008 in this role he lectured and presented to more than 20,000 fellow fitness professionals and students.

Steve played a key role in the development of the training systems and launch of two significant products in the fitness industry: the Reebok Deck and Reebok Core Board®. As a personal trainer, in addition to teaching the teachers and working with the rich and famous he has been involved in the training of many international athletes and sports personalities at Liverpool FC, Arsenal FC, Manchester Utd FC, the Welsh RFU, and UK athletics.

Within the fitness industry he has acted as a consultant to leading brand names, including Nestlé, Kelloggs, Reebok and Adidas.

His media experience includes being guest expert for the BBC and writing for numerous publications including *The Times*, *The Independent*, *The Daily Telegraph*, *Runner's World*, *Men's Fitness*, *Rugby News*, *Health & Fitness*, *Zest*, *Ultra-FIT*, *Men's Health UK* and *Australia* and many more.

Steve's expertise is the development of logical, user friendly, safe and effective training programmes. The work that he is most proud of, however, isn't his celebrity projects, but the changes to ordinary people's lives that never get reported.

Now that he has been teaching fitness throughout his 20s, 30s and now 40s, he has developed a tremendous ability to relate to the challenges that people face to incorporate exercise into their lifestyle, and while the fitness industry expects personal trainers to work with clients for a short period of time, Steve has been working with many of his clients for nearly two decades, continuously evolving to meet their changing needs.

His fun and direct approach has resulted in many couch potatoes running out of excuses and transforming into fitness converts.

www.Trade-Secrets-of-a-Personal-Trainer.com

index